P9-ECU-518

AROMATHERAPY

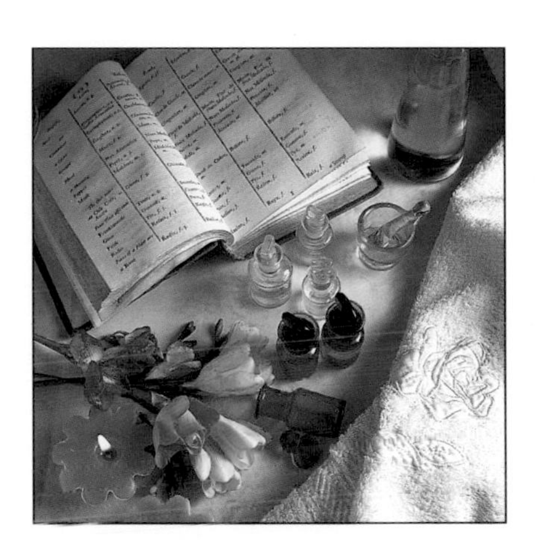

ANNA SELBY

PETER ALBRIGHT, M.D., SERIES EDITOR

MACMILLAN • USA

A QUARTO BOOK

MACMILLAN
A Simon and Schuster Macmillan Company
1633 Broadway
New York, NY 10019-6785

ISBN 0-02-860832-1

The book was designed and produced by
Quarto Inc.
The Old Brewery
6 Blundell Street
London N7 9BH

Senior editor Sally MacEachern
Editor Alison Leach
Editorial assistant Judith Evans
Indexer Dorothy Frame
Senior art editor Penny Cobb
Designers Alyson Kyles, Sarah Pollack
Picture researcher Susannah Jayes
Illustrator Graham Berry
Photographers Laura Wickenden, Martin Norris
Models Tim Donelly, Kate Mitchell
Picture research manager Giulia Hetherington
Editorial director Mark Dartford
Art director Moira Clinch

Typeset by Central Southern Typesetters, Eastbourne
Manufactured in Hong Kong by Regent Publishing Services Ltd
Printed in China by Leefung-Asco Printers Ltd

10 9 8 7 6 5 4 3 2 1

CONTENTS

INTRODUCTION 4

THE ESSENTIAL OILS 8

Relaxing Starter Pack 9

Theraputic Starter Pack 12

First Aid 15

Children's Starter Pack 16

Other Oils 17

BASIC TECHNIQUES 20

Using the Oils 22

Massage Basics 24

The Basic Massage Strokes 26

Full Body Massage 29

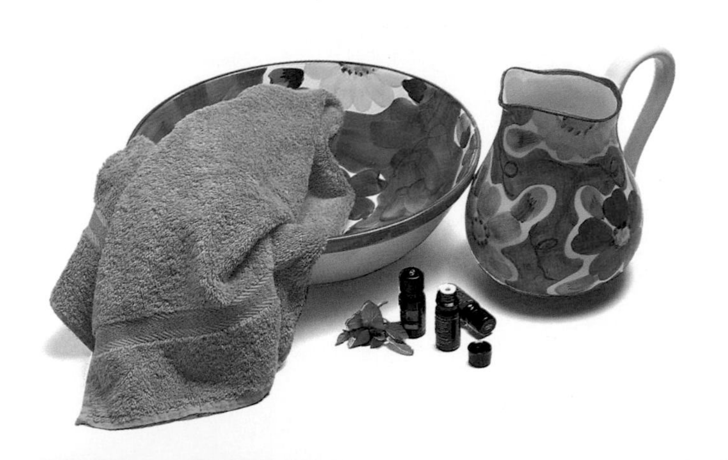

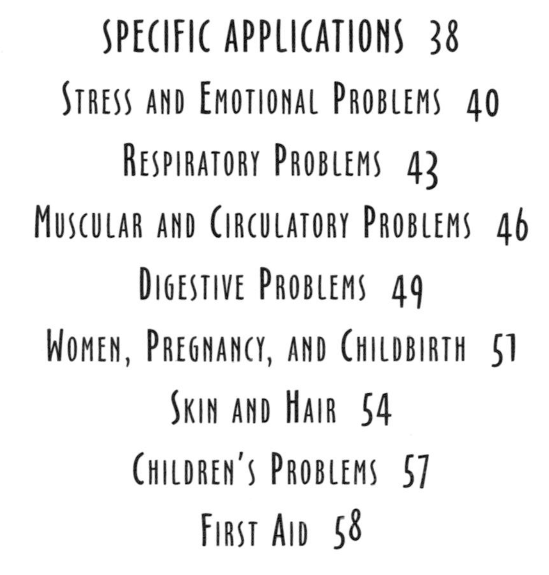

SPECIFIC APPLICATIONS 38

Stress and Emotional Problems 40

Respiratory Problems 43

Muscular and Circulatory Problems 46

Digestive Problems 49

Women, Pregnancy, and Childbirth 51

Skin and Hair 54

Children's Problems 57

First Aid 58

CONSULTING AN AROMATHERAPIST 60

Useful Addresses 61

Reading List 61

Index 62

Acknowledgments 64

INTRODUCTION

Aromatherapy is, as its name suggests, a therapy that uses aromas. These aromas are produced from many different plants – flowers, trees, and herbs – and from various parts of those plants – roots, leaves, flowers, bark, and rind. The volatile essential oil of the plant (including its odor) – often referred to as the plant's "life-force" – is captured through a process of extraction or distillation. Using plants for healing is, of course, a practice that began with our most distant ancestors, who ate them, made infusions to drink, or applied them to the skin. They were also burned as incense in rituals, and in ancient Egypt, Greece, and Rome, fragrances from plants (though not actual distilled essences) were used for medicinal and cosmetic purposes and very highly valued.

The essences of such plants as eucalyptus, rosemary, and geranium are extracted for use as aromatherapy oils.

When the tomb of Tutankhamen was opened in 1922, there was still a lingering fragrance of frankincense from the pots placed there over 3,000 years before. And, of course, frankincense and myrrh – which produce two of the most powerful essences in common use – were offered by the Magi, the three wise men, to the infant Jesus. This gives some measure of the value given them in the ancient world.

The distillation of essential oils, as now known, however, is thought to have been discovered in the late tenth century by the Arab physician known in the West as Avicenna. The process was brought back to the West by the Crusaders and applied to our native plants. Although the use of essential oils as a therapy flourished for a while, it had virtually disappeared by the beginning of the twentieth century. Then in the 1920s, René-Maurice Gattefosse, a French chemist, became interested in essential oils and discovered that not only were they powerful antiseptics, they also had remarkable healing powers. He learned this from personal experience. When his hand was severely burned in an experiment in his laboratory, he

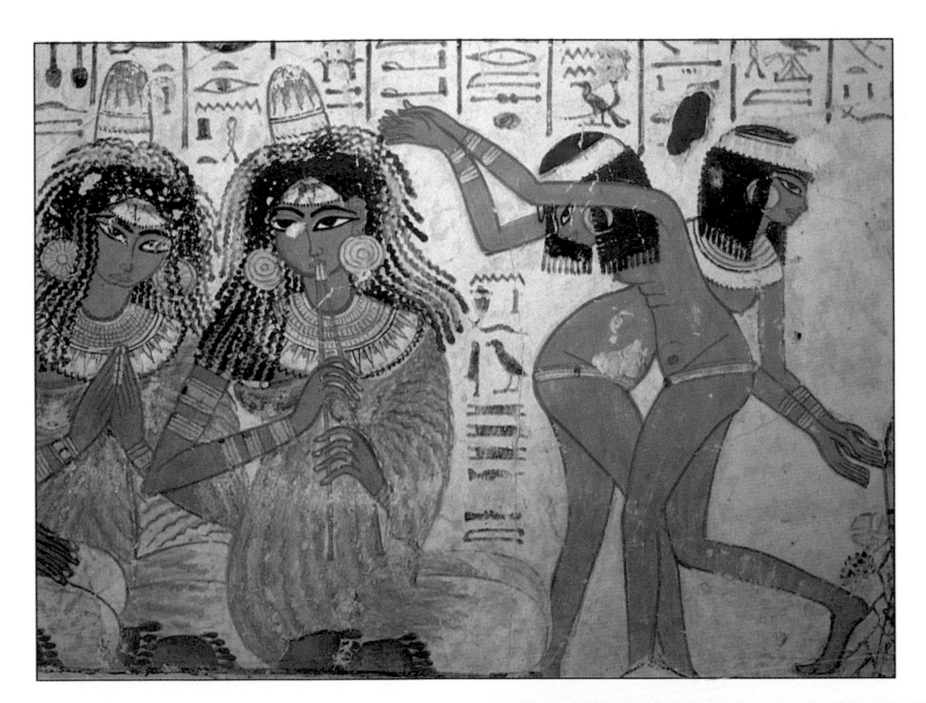

In ancient Egypt plant extracts were used as medicine, cosmetics, and for ritual purposes.

plunged it into pure lavender oil. Not only did it heal remarkably quickly, there was no infection and no scar. Hardly surprisingly, he continued his investigations and in 1928 wrote the book that coined the name by which the therapy has been known ever since, *Aromathérapie*.

The first English book on the subject, *The Art of Aromatherapy*, by Robert Tisserand, was not published until 1977, and it is only since then that interest in aromatherapy has really begun to take hold in the English-speaking world. Since then, aromatherapy has played a part in the remarkable resurgence of natural medicine. Holistic medicine emphasizes treating the whole person (mind, body, and spirit) rather than mere symptoms; using non-invasive, natural techniques; and taking responsibility for our own health. Obviously, aromatherapy embodies all these principles.

Although the oils can be used in a wide variety of ways, aromatherapy is very much linked with massage. A massage from a skilled aromatherapist is a real treat and deeply relaxing – making a good antidote to the high levels of stress that abound today. Depending upon the blend of oils used, the massage can also affect specific problems (see pages 38-59), as diverse as headaches and menstrual cramps, a sports injury, or indigestion. A massage with essential oils also involves the use of both of the pathways into the body that they can take – via the skin and via the olfactory system.

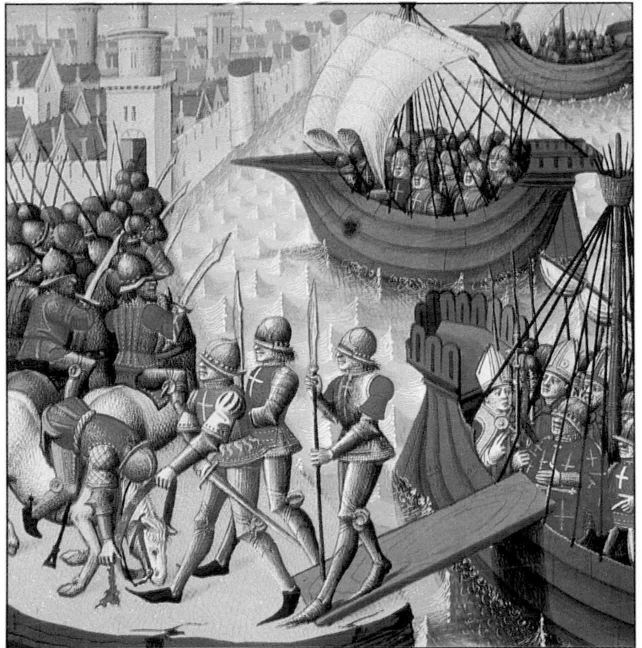

The distillation of essential oils is believed to have started with the Arab physician, Avicenna. The process was brought to the West by the Crusaders.

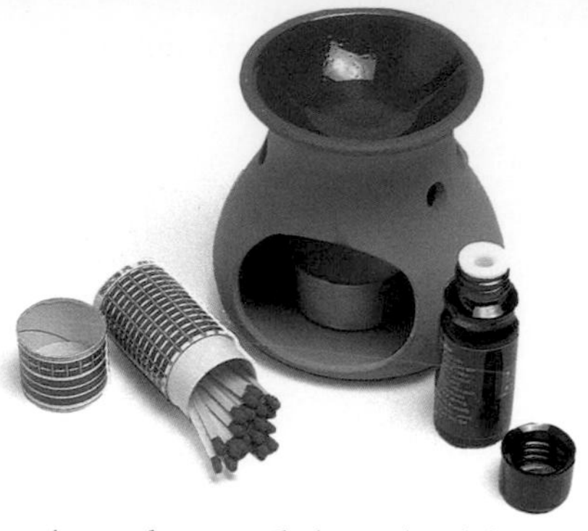

Aromatherapy oils have the ability to affect our moods and fill a whole room with their fragrance on a simple burner.

The Olfactory System

The sense of smell is today undervalued to the extent that it is generally regarded as the least of the senses. Yet research has shown that people respond to smell on an emotional level more strongly than to the other senses. A scent can trigger a whole string of half-forgotten memories – the area of the brain associated with smell is the same as that of the memory. Certain oils also have a remarkable ability to transform and balance our emotions – relieving anxiety, depression, or mental fatigue.

It is thought that the effect of smell is so strong and so immediate because the olfactory nerve is in direct contact with the limbic system, the emotional center of the brain. The olfactory nerve cells terminate in the cilia, the tiny hairs in the nasal cavity. Their response to the stimulus of an aroma is to transmit a direct impulse to that part of the brain where the memory and emotions lie and connect to the hypothalamus and the pituitary gland that governs our hormonal systems. While a great deal more research on how the sense of smell works is still needed, there can be little doubt that its effect on both mind and body is profound.

Skin Absorption

During massage, when essential oils are dissolved in a carrier oil (or in the bathwater), they can be absorbed through the skin via the hair follicles into the bloodstream or lymphatic system and then circulated throughout the body. The oils have a generally stabilizing effect on the body: lowering high blood pressure, stimulating sluggish circulation, and promoting detoxification and healthy cell renewal. (For the therapeutic actions of specific oils, see pages 9–19).

How to Get Started

This book is primarily about self-help – but see page 60 for information on consulting a professional aromatherapist. You can buy the oils from reputable health food stores or via mail order (page 61). It is important to realize that these oils are very potent. Use them only in the dilutions given in this book and remember to check the warning list of oils to avoid in various circumstances (page 39). This is particularly necessary if you are pregnant or using the oils on babies or children.

Never try to treat serious conditions yourself. Essential oils have their limitations, and you should always consult a qualified medical practitioner if you think you have any cause for concern.

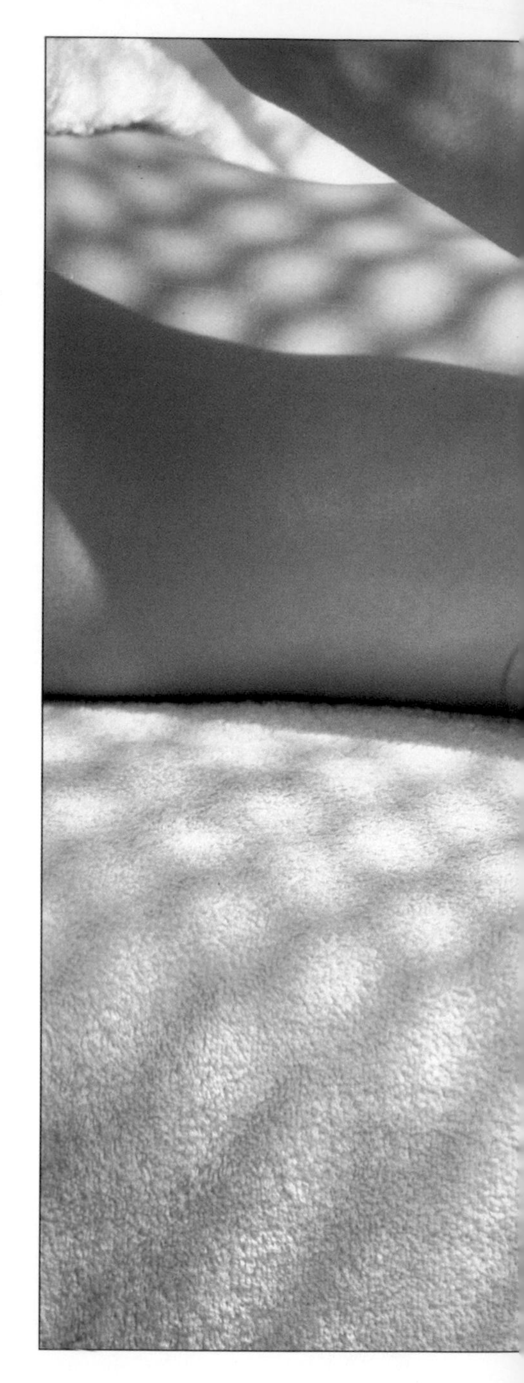

An aromatherapy massage is deeply relaxing, and the oils can penetrate the body both through the skin and by inhalation via the olfactory system.

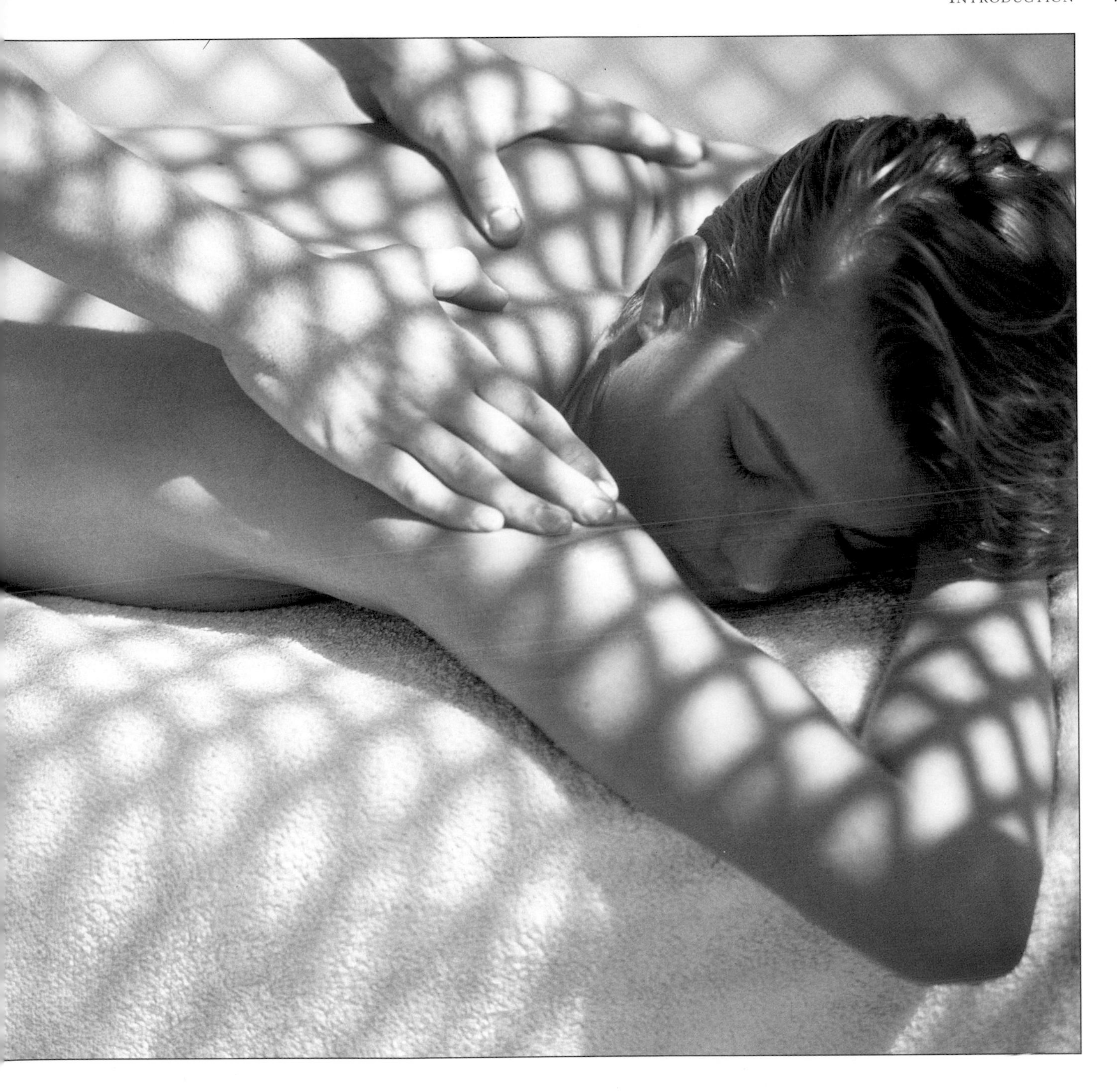

THE ESSENTIAL OILS

The essential oils used in aromatherapy come from a wide variety of natural sources — herbs, flowers, leaves, wood, resin, seeds, fruit rind, roots, and gum. They are extracted using a number of methods, often by steam distillation, to form a pure, highly volatile oil. There are other oils on the market, often described as "scented with essential oils," which are definitely not to be confused with the real thing. True essential oils are undiluted and come in small dark blue or brown bottles.

Aromatherapy oils can be used on many levels — physical, emotional, mental, and spiritual — whether on their own, inhaled from a tissue, or in conjunction with other therapies. It is important to dilute them before use (see dilution chart on page 22).

Warning

- Except in the rare instances specifically mentioned in this book, essential oils should not be taken internally or applied undiluted directly to the skin.
- Citrus oils — bergamot, lemon, orange, mandarin, and so on — should never be used on the skin before exposure to the sun as they may cause irritation.
- Keep oils out of the reach of children and, if they are accidentally swallowed, do not induce vomiting, but seek urgent medical help.
- There are several contra-indications to be considered (see the box on page 39 before using any oils).

There are several essential oils boxes on the market in which to store your oils. Alternatively, you can keep them in the fridge with their tops tightly sealed (or they may flavor the food).

RELAXING STARTER PACK

Aromatherapy oils are perhaps best known for their powers to balance and lift the spirits. These euphoric essences can be effective for all sorts of emotional problems, from stress and fatigue to depression and premenstrual syndrome (PMS). There are a number of ways they can be used for such treatments, but probably the best is as a full body massage (see pages 24-37). They can also be used as room scents on vaporizers, in the bath water, or simply inhaled from pillow or a tissue. The 11 essences listed here are those most readily available and easy to use. Other oils that can be used in this category are peppermint and bergamot (see pages 13 and 16), melissa, patchouli, and orange (see pages 17-19).

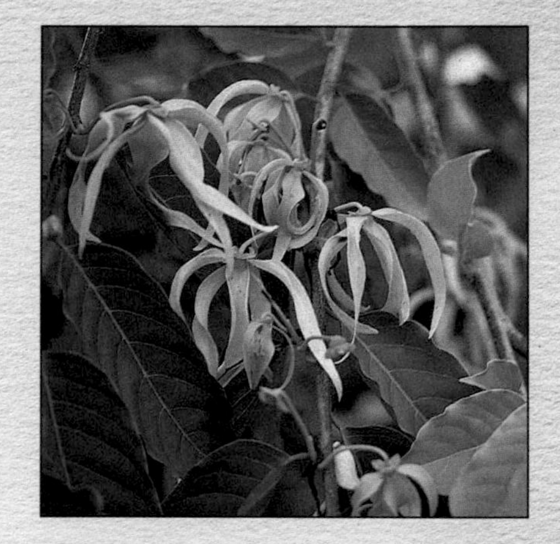

Ylang-ylang *(above)*
(Cananga odorata)
Distilled from the flowers of the tropical ylang-ylang tree, this heady oil is renowned as an antidepressant and aphrodisiac. Its sweet, exotic scent makes it a popular ingredient in many perfumes, but it can be quite overpowering – only a few drops should be used in a blend with other oils, particularly jasmine, bergamot, and rose, as the strong scent may otherwise cause a headache.

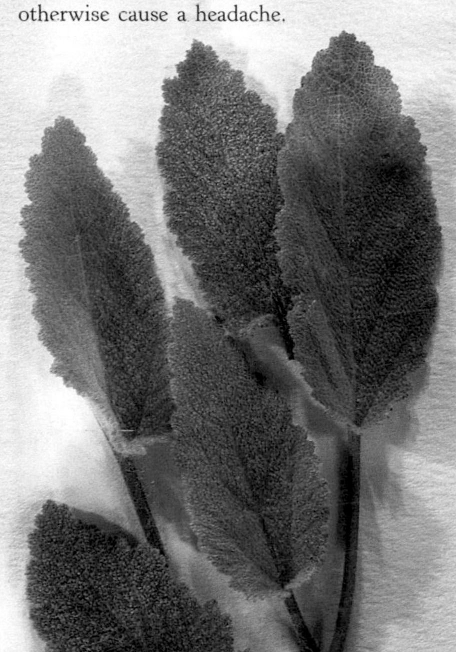

Neroli
(Citrus aurantium)
This oil is also known as orange blossom, and it is extracted from the flowers of the orange tree (see also Orange and Petitgrain). Like rose, it is both one of the most expensive oils and one of the most feminine. It is both calming and uplifting, and very valuable as an antidepressant, especially in cases of nervous tension, extreme anxiety, hysteria, and shock. It also has a generally calming effect on the heart and is good for palpitations. It combines well with woody and other floral essences.
OTHER USES: Insomnia; most skin conditions; as a facial toner, especially for mature skin.

Clary sage (*left*)
(Salvia sclarea)
Clary sage is not to be confused with sage, which is a more toxic essential oil best left to professional aromatherapists. Clary sage, however, is generally non-toxic, *though it should be avoided during pregnancy*. It is extremely euphoric and so is very good as an antidepressant. In fact, it has quite an intoxicating effect and so should never be used on someone who has been drinking! It blends well with sandalwood and lavender, and has rather a sweet scent. It is safe to use for children and has a very calming effect on them, too, if mixed into a bath.
OTHER USES: As a general tonic and sedative; for menstrual problems, both cramps and scanty, irregular periods.

Geranium *(below)*
(Pelargonium odorantissimum/graveolens)
The sweet scent of this oil is strong, but fresh rather than cloying, and it blends well with a very wide range of other oils, including lavender, rose, patchouli, neroli, and bergamot. It has antidepressant and sedative properties, and is good for anxiety, stress, and mood swings.
OTHER USES: Many skin problems, including eczema and acne; throat infections; diarrhea; burns; as an insect repellant. Safe for children.

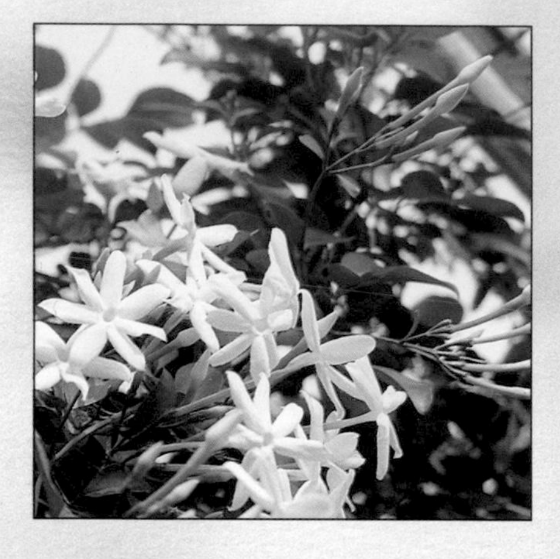

Jasmine *(above)*
(Jasminum officinale)
Jasmine is one of the most powerful of the antidepressant oils. It has an exquisitely sweet floral fragrance which blends with other oils such as rose, clary sage, and the citrus oils. It is another expensive oil. In addition to being an antidepressant, it has aphrodisiac and sedative properties. It should be used only in moderation – both in terms of quantity in a blend (usually two or three drops are sufficient) and frequency.
OTHER USES: Coughs and catarrh; female reproductive problems, especially labor pains, to increase breast milk, and for postnatal depression.

Vetivert
(Andropogen muricatus)
Vetivert is traditionally associated with men's toiletries, and its woody, smoky aroma contrasts with many of the more flowery scents of the relaxing oils – making this a good one to use if you are going to give a massage to a man. Vetivert comes from a tall, scented grass and has a deeply relaxing effect. It is ideal for use in a bath or for massage, where it blends well with lavender.

Lemon *(below)*
(Citrus limon)
Lemon is a very refreshing, cleansing oil, and this uplifting quality can be useful for depression and fatigue. The oil comes from the peel of the fruit and has a very distinctive citrus smell that combines well with, among others, bergamot, geranium, ginger, eucalyptus, and juniper. Besides its emotionally clarifying properties, the oil is renowned, like lemon juice, for strengthening the immune system, particularly against colds, fever, flu, and infections. *Lemon oil is phototoxic – do not use on the skin before exposure to sunlight.*
OTHER USES: Sinusitis; asthma; brittle nails; insect bites. It has also been suggested that it can dissolve kidney stones.

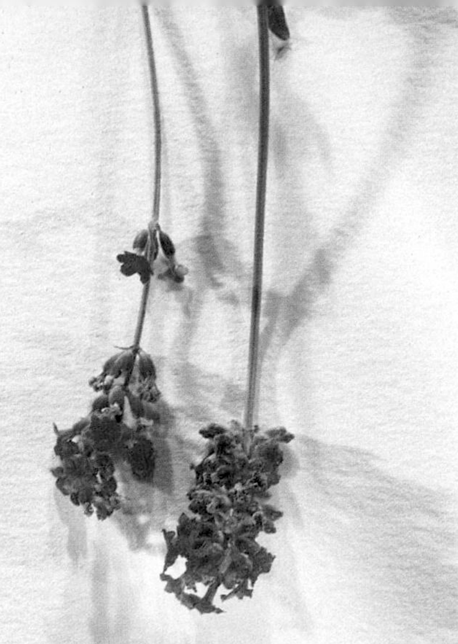

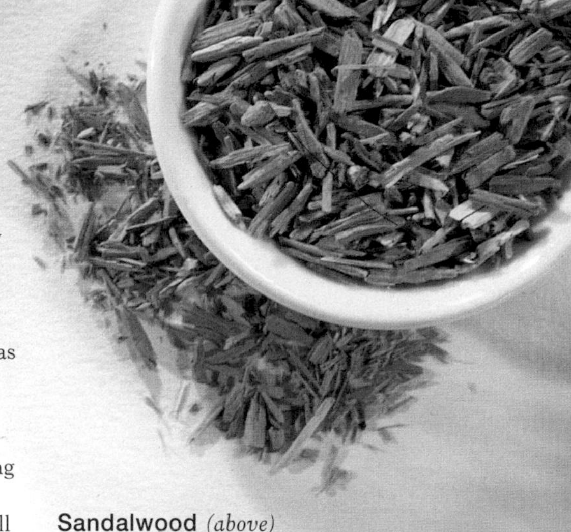

Rose
Rosa damascena **(damask rose)**
Rosa centifolia **(cabbage rose)**
The rose has been prized since antiquity for its healing and regenerative powers. Its scent is, of course, heady and very feminine, and it is commonly linked in aromatherapy to female problems, such as regulating menstrual periods. It is strongly antidepressant and aphrodisiac, and works well for most emotional problems with its stabilizing and uplifting qualities. It blends well with most other flower essences. It works particularly well in skin preparations and is even said to have powers of rejuvenation! It is one of the gentlest oils, and its stabilizing effect works equally well on the heart and circulation as well as headaches. It is one of the most expensive oils, but as it has such a powerful aroma, a little goes a long way.
OTHER USES: Headache; eczema; hayfever; as an antiseptic. Safe for children.

Lavender *(above)*
(Lavandula officinalis/angustifolia)
If you had to choose just one oil that would suit every circumstance to take with you to a desert island, it would almost certainly be lavender. This versatile oil is derived from the flowers of the herb and has a familiar fresh scent, often used in perfume. It is one of the safest essences to use – even for children – and one of the few that can be used directly on the skin without being blended in carrier oil. It is both antiseptic and healing, particularly on burns (where it promotes skin regeneration), bites, and stings. It blends extremely well with most other oils (especially floral or citrus) and has strong sedative and calming properties, making it very effective for problems such as tension, depression, and insomnia.
OTHER USES: Headaches; skin problems; high blood pressure; respiratory and digestive disorders; cystitis; sunburn. It is useful for any inflammatory condition, as a painkiller, and as an antiseptic.

Basil *(right)*
(Ocimum basilicum)
Basil is one of the most uplifting oils and works especially well with emotional problems connected with anxiety and mental fatigue. Used in the bath or simply inhaled from a tissue, it gives an instant boost – concentrating the mind and strengthening confidence. It is also quite a powerful antiseptic and is excellent for respiratory problems such as bronchitis, colds, coughs, and sinusitis. It blends well with clary sage, bergamot, and geranium. *It should, however, be used only in moderation and never during pregnancy.*
OTHER USES: Muscular aches and pains; rheumatism; as an insect repellant.

Sandalwood *(above)*
(Santalum album)
This warm, sweet, woody essence comes from the tropical sandalwood tree and has been known in the East for its medicinal, cosmetic, and embalming properties for thousands of years. It has a calming, anti-depressant effect and is also said to have aphrodisiac properties. Many men find it more appealing than the more flowery essences. It combines well with such resonating scents as rose and neroli, and is an important constituent in many perfumes.
OTHER USES: For the respiratory system, especially sore throats and laryngitis; insomnia; diarrhea; as a diuretic; for dry skin.

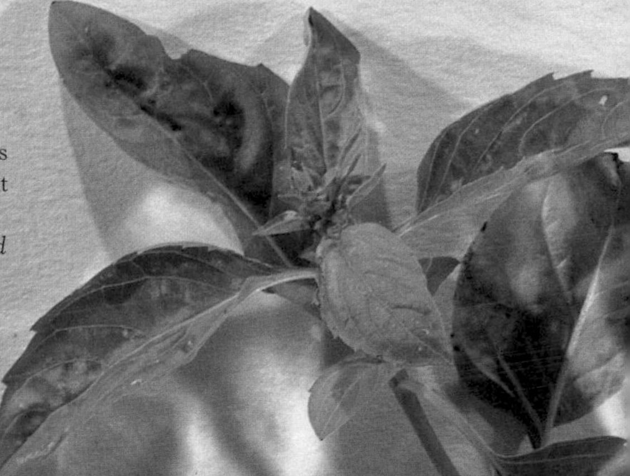

Therapeutic Starter Pack

Essential oils can be very effective in treating certain conditions. While it would be foolish to suggest they can be used exclusively to cure a whole range of medical problems, they are often able, within their limitations, to give relief to people suffering from such conditions as rheumatism and arthritis, back pain, respiratory problems, and a variety of minor ailments. This starter-pack of 11 oils does not include such delicious fragrances as those found in the relaxing starter pack. However, they can be mixed with some of them, the most important of which is lavender. The therapeutic properties of this oil are on a par with its relaxing ones. Other oils with strongly therapeutic powers include clary sage, sandalwood, and lemon (pages 9-11); camomile (page 16); and tea tree, fennel, and marjoram (page 15).

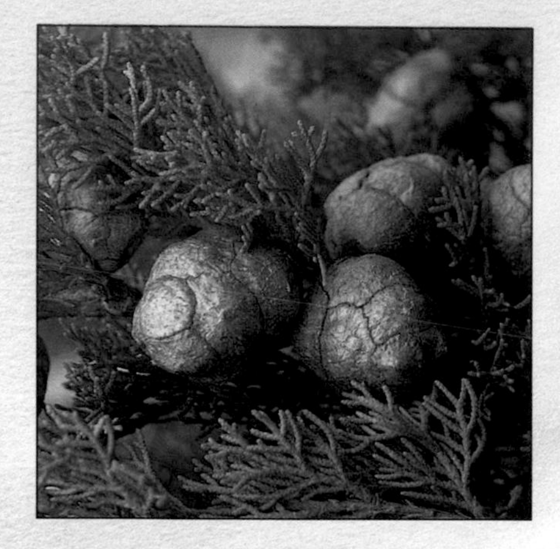

Cypress *(above)*
(Cupressus sempervirens)
The smoky, woody aroma of cypress has a very soothing effect and so is very useful for anxiety and insomnia. It has a remarkable ability to staunch the flow of blood and is excellent for stopping nose bleeds. It is very helpful for varicose veins (though it may only prevent the worsening of the condition, as opposed to curing it), hemorrhoids, and oily skin. It blends well with cedarwood, lavender, clary sage, and citrus oils.
OTHER USES: Cellulite; spasmodic coughing and bronchitis; swollen joints; wounds.

Bergamot
(Citrus bergamia)
The essential oil does not come from the herb called bergamot, but from the fruit of the bergamot tree. It is extracted from the rind of the fruit, which resembles a small orange, so it has a fresh, sweet citrus smell. Its uplifting, refreshing quality gives it as much value as a relaxing oil (for depression, anxiety, and stress) as a therapeutic one. It is excellent as an antiseptic, notably on a vaporizer against airborne infections. It is also very effective for skin problems such as acne, eczema, and psoriasis, *but should not be used on skin before exposure to sunlight.*
OTHER USES: As an insect repellant and on insect bites; sore throats, halitosis, tonsillitis; cystitis, and thrush.

Ginger *(below)*
(Zingiber officinale)
Ginger is noted for its warming qualities and so is particularly effective for respiratory problems. Used sparingly in a blend with oils such as lemon, cilantro, and patchouli, it has a stimulating, effect. This makes it useful for all sorts of muscular aches and pains, arthritis, rheumatism, sprains, and poor circulation. *It should not be used on the skin before exposure to sunlight.*
OTHER USES: Nausea and travel sickness; constipation.

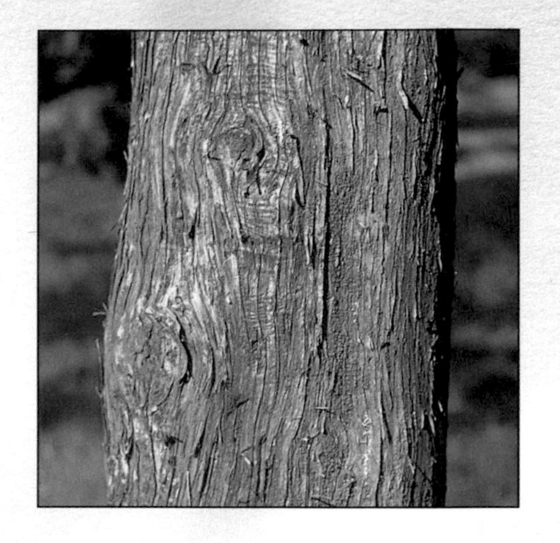

Cedarwood *(above)*
(Juniperus virginiana)
The oil from the Virginia cedar has a smell which inevitably reminds one of pencils, as this is its principal product. The ancient Egyptians, however, prized the cedar of Lebanon as an ingredient for mummification and cosmetics. It is excellent for respiratory problems, such as bronchitis, catarrh, and coughs. Its other principal use is in skin complaints such as eczema and dermatitis. It blends well with sandalwood, cypress, juniper, rose, and patchouli. *Do not use during pregnancy.*
OTHER USES: Cystitis; dandruff, oily hair and skin; as an insect repellant.

Frankincense
(Boswellia thurifera)
The high value of frankincense in the ancient world is reflected in it being one of the three gifts offered to the baby Jesus. It has certain similarities to myrrh, one of the other gifts, but has a warmer, lighter, sweet fragrance. It is useful for rheumatism and arthritis, cystitis and menstrual problems, and as an inhalant for catarrh, laryngitis, and bronchitis. Blend with lavender, sandalwood, rose, bergamot, neroli, and other spices.
OTHER USES: Anxiety and stress.
It has also been prized for thousands of years as a rejuvenator for dry, mature skin and is said to stimulate cell renewal.

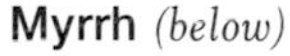

Myrrh *(below)*
*(Commiphora myrrha/
Balsamodendron myrrha)*
Myrrh shares many of the characteristics and properties of frankincense, though it has a slightly more musky, bitter smell and a more strengthening therapeutic effect. It is particularly useful for canker sores and for healing cuts and wounds. Like frankincense, it is thought to be good for the complexion. It blends with other woody, spicy oils such as frankincense, sandalwood, cedarwood, and ginger. *It should never be used in pregnancy.*
OTHER USES: Coughs, colds and bronchitis; stretch marks; yeast.

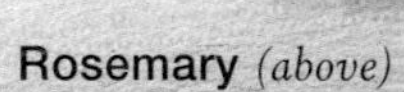

Rosemary *(above)*
(Rosmarinus officinalis)
In addition to being an excellent antiseptic, rosemary has a generally warming, stimulating, and balancing effect on all the internal organs. It has a similar effect on the mind to that of basil – invigorating and strengthening. It is particularly useful for rheumatism, arthritis, and general muscular aches and pains. It is traditionally used in many hair preparations. It combines well with other herbal oils and cedarwood. *Do not use during pregnancy.*
OTHER USES: Coughs, colds, and flu.

Juniper
(Juniperus communis)
Juniper is a diuretic and very effective for urinary infections and fluid retention, especially during menstruation. It is the most powerful ingredient in the recipe on page 51 for cystitis, and in expelling uric acid from the joints, it is also useful for rheumatism, arthritis, and gout. It stimulates the circulation, purifies the bloodstream, and acts on the kidneys. It is also excellent for indigestion and flatulence. It blends well with lavender, cypress, rosemary, and cedarwood. Use only the oil made from the berry, not that from the wood. *It should not be used during pregnancy, nor for those with kidney disease.*

Benzoin
(Styrax benzoin)
Benzoin used to be known as gum benjamin, and it is made from the gum of the tropical benzoin tree. It is one of the most familiar of incense smells. It has an overall warming effect, and when mixed with other oils and used as an inhalant, it is excellent for colds, coughs, bronchitis, and flu – all conditions that respond to its warming properties. It is also beneficial for urinary infections, such as cystitis, and for skin problems such as dermatitis. It blends well with sandalwood.
Other uses: For rheumatism and arthritis, as a compress; as a general sedative.

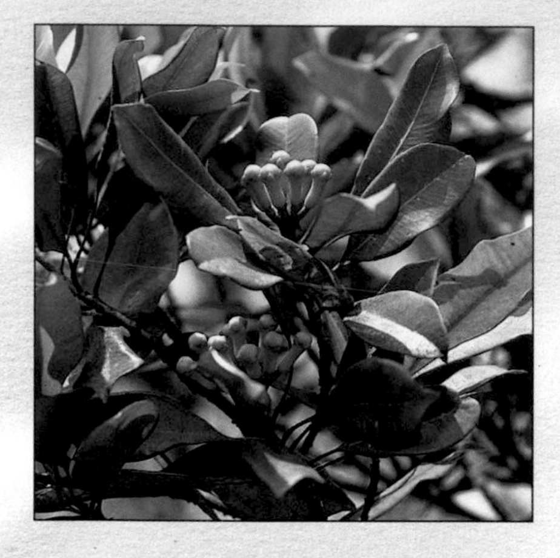

Clove *(above)*
(Syzygium aromaticum)
The spicy smell of clove is familiar from its widespread use in cooking. It has long been associated with relief from toothache, though it can also be used (one or two drops in a blend with other oils, such as rose, bergamot, and lavender) as a compress for wounds, bruises, and burns. There are various types of clove oil – made from the leaf, stem, or bud. For home use, always use the clove bud oil, as the others can cause skin irritation.
Other uses: Arthritis and rheumatism; as part of a steam inhalation for bronchitis; as a mosquito repellant.

Eucalyptus *(below)*
(Eucalyptus globulus)
Eucalyptus has a good deal in common with basil oil and delivers the same boost to the system, energizing and invigorating mind and body. Its distinctive aroma is well known from its use in OTC decongestant medicines for colds. It is an extremely powerful natural antiseptic, and a few drops on the pillow or a vaporizer can often ward off potential colds and infections. It can be blended with lemon, lavender, pine, and cypress.
Other uses: Rheumatism and arthritis; cystitis (use in bath); cold sores; headaches; all respiratory disorders; against infection.

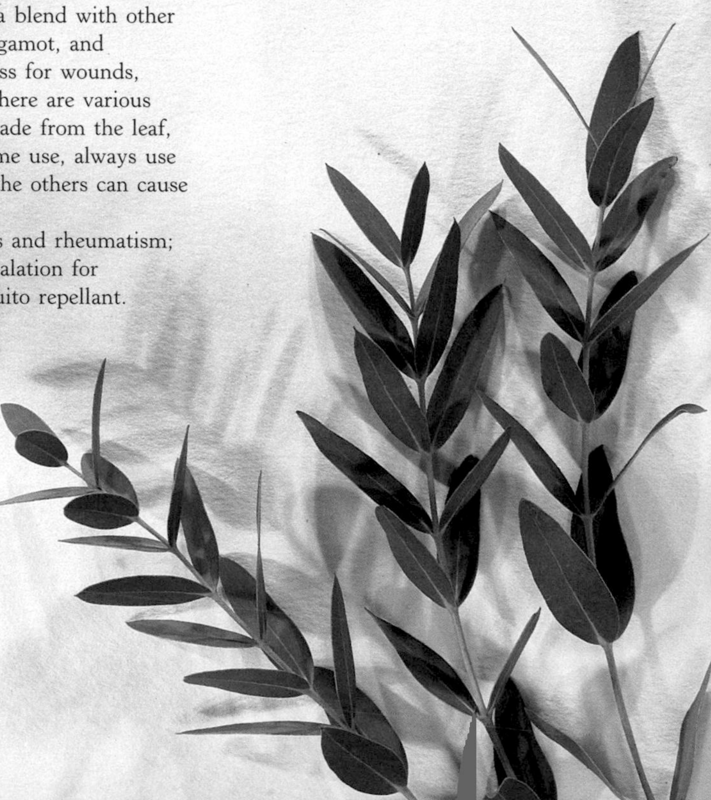

First Aid

There are a number of multi-purpose oils that make up an ideal first aid kit to deal with minor emergencies, to be used either at home or to take on vacation. As always, lavender is indispensable (see page 9) – it can be used directly on the skin and has excellent soothing, healing, and antiseptic properties. It is also a stabilizing and uplifting oil on an emotional level and is good at dispelling headaches and relieving insomnia. Eucalyptus, rosemary, and peppermint arc also very useful in the medicine cabinet, between them treating a wide variety of ailments from colds to indigestion. Two other emergency essentials are not aromatherapy oils, but to be highly recommended nonetheless. One is arnica cream or ointment which has an outstanding ability to prevent bruising. The other is a Bach flower remedy, "Rescue Remedy," which is ideal in cases of shock and trauma.

Tea tree
(Melaleuca alternifolia)
This remarkable oil comes from an Australian tree, and while the essence is a comparative newcomer to aromatherapy, it has been used by Australian aborigines for many years. It is an extremely useful therapeutic oil and a prodigious antiseptic. It soothes and heals wounds and is useful against skin infections, canker sores, cystitis, insect bites and stings, blisters and burns, spots and acne, diaper rash, and fungal infections like athlete's foot and ringworm. It fights off colds, coughs, sore throats, herpes, and flu, and eases diarrhea. It also soothes sunburn and is an effective insect repellant. It blends well with lavender, clary sage, rosemary, marjoram, and geranium.
OTHER USES: Yeast, bronchitis.

Marjoram *(right)*
(Origanum majorana)
This familiar culinary herb produces a woody aroma with a warming, comforting quality. The oil is very effective against bruising and for soothing sprains, strains, and general muscular aches and pains. It is excellent massaged into the temples to alleviate headache and migraine, and has a calming effect emotionally, making it useful against insomnia and tension. It is also renowned for alleviating period cramps and PMS, constipation, flatulence, and indigestion. It mixes well with other herbal oils, tea tree, and eucalyptus. *It should not be used during pregnancy.*
OTHER USES: High blood pressure; colds and bronchitis; rheumatism and arthritis.

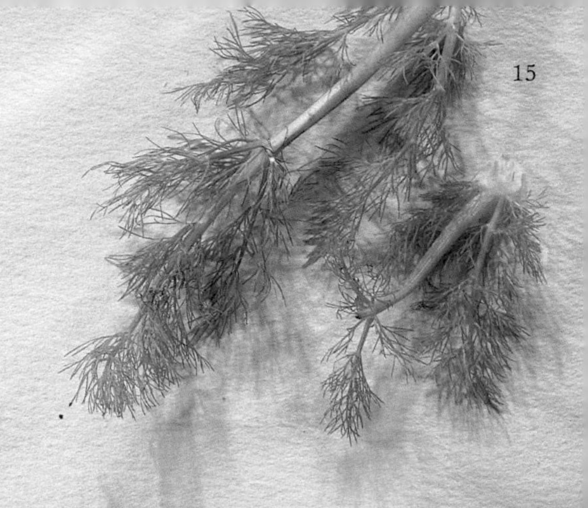

Fennel *(above)*
(Foeniculum vulgare)
Fennel is another well-known culinary herb, and its essential oil is noted for its calming and toning effects on the digestive system. This means it is particularly good in cases of nausea and vomiting, colic, constipation, flatulence, and even hiccups. It is also used as a diuretic and for dissolving kidney stones. Traditionally, it is supposed to increase a mother's milk. It blends well with geranium, lavender, and sandalwood. *It should not be used during pregnancy or by epileptics.*
OTHER USES: Bruising; cellulite; obesity; asthma; bronchitis.

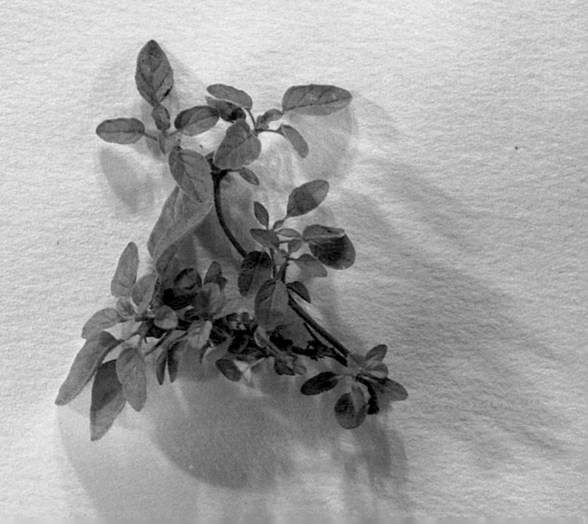

Children's Starter Pack

A starter pack of aromatherapy oils is particularly useful for children – few mothers want to subject babies and young children to drugs and antibiotics and their possible side-effects, if they can avoid it. Any essences to be used for children must, of course, be very gentle ones, and *you should only use the ones mentioned here or on page 57.* Yet again, lavender is one of the most useful oils – it is very gentle, soothing, and healing, and effective against everything from sleeplessness to diaper rash. It can be applied undiluted even to a child's delicate skin. Other useful oils for children include geranium, rose, and clary sage (pages 10-11); eucalyptus (page 14), and tea tree (page 15).

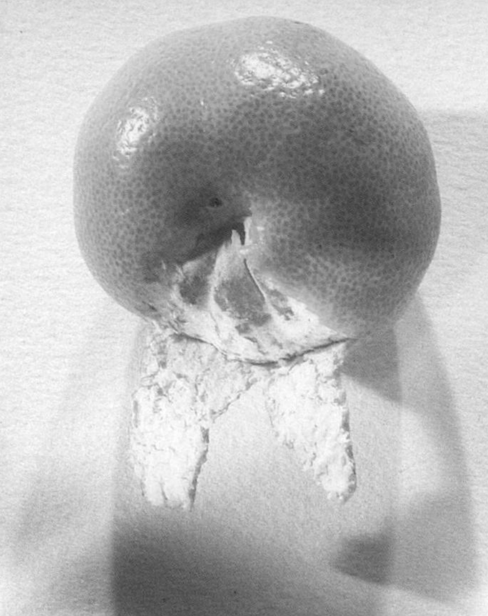

Mandarin *(above)*
(Citrus reticulata)
The very sweet citrus smell of this oil and its gentle, soothing properties make it ideal for children. It blends well with geranium and is good for hiccups, stomach upsets, insomnia, and for calming down overexcited or tearful children, as it has the dual ability of simultaneously calming and lifting the spirits.
OTHER USES: To prevent stretch marks in pregnancy; fluid retention; obesity; for digestive and liver problems in the elderly.

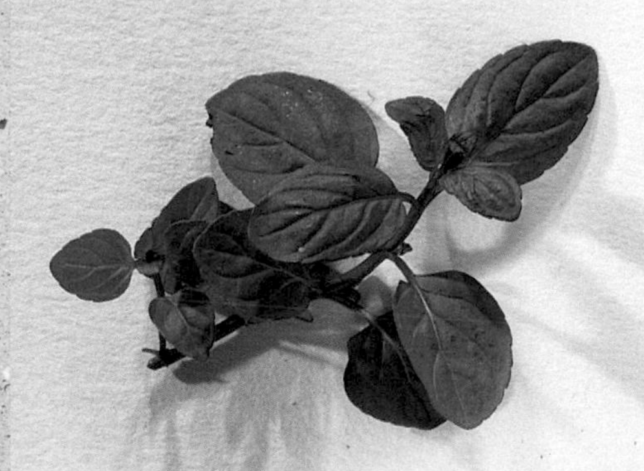

Camomile
(Anthemis nobilis /Roman camomile)
(Matricaria chamomilla /German camomile)
With lavender, camomile is probably the most important essential oil for children. It is extremely gentle and calming while at the same time being antiseptic, anti-inflammatory, and antispasmodic. This makes it ideal for a very wide variety of childhood ailments from teething pain, earache, colic, vomiting, and diarrhea to convulsions, tantrums, and sleeplessness. It can be used on diaper rash, burns, and scalds. It is very soothing blended with lavender, rose, geranium, or clary sage in the bath or as a massage oil.
OTHER USES: Acne and eczema; rheumatism and arthritis; muscular aches and pains.

Peppermint *(left)*
(Mentha piperita)
Peppermint oil has a strong, distinctive smell and is more suitable for older than for very young children. It is useful in relieving toothache (applied on a cotton swab directly to the teeth) and for nausea and travel sickness. It is good for older children's stomachaches and for colds and flu. It is an excellent antiseptic, and as it has sedative qualities, it can have a quite calming, soothing effect on over-excited children. It relieves itchiness of the skin to help soothe chickenpox symptoms. It blends well with lavender and eucalyptus.
OTHER USES: Headache and migraine; bronchitis; sinusitis; palpitations; ringworm and scabies.

OTHER OILS

Besides the oils mentioned in the starter packs, many more essences are available that are suitable for home use. There are still others that have ambiguous or toxic properties which make them difficult for the non-professional to use. Those listed here are safe and effective for home use unless otherwise indicated. Some act as substitutes for more common or more expensive oils, while others have curative powers over very specific ailments.

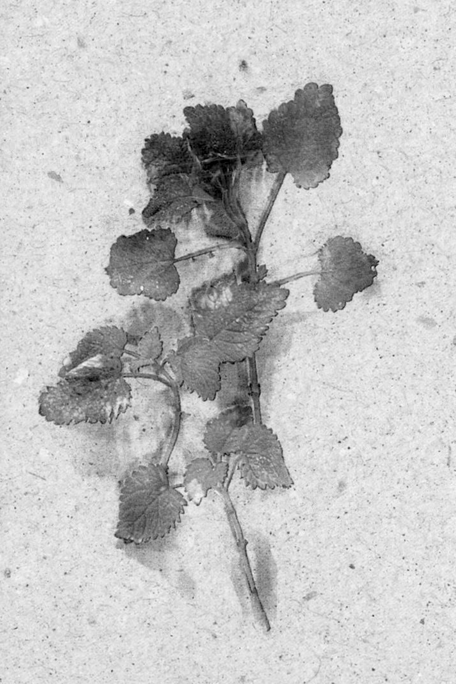

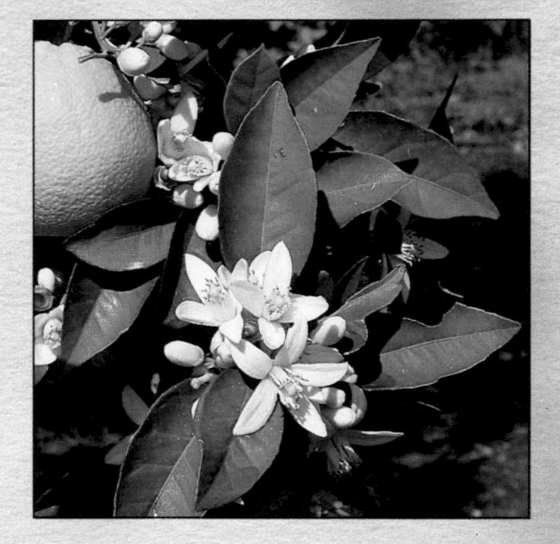

Petitgrain *(above)*
(Citrus aurantium)
This is one of the three essences to come from the orange tree, this one from the leaf. Petitgrain has a good deal in common with neroli, which comes from the blossom of the tree. It has a fresh, uplifting flowery aroma and is frequently used in hair and skin care. It is also a natural deodorant.
OTHER USES: Insomnia; nervous exhaustion.

Melissa (Lemon balm) *(left)*
(Melissa officinalis)
This gentle, soothing essence balances the emotions and acts as a general tonic – on the heart, the nervous system, and the menstrual cycle (where it regulates the periods and soothes menstrual pain). On an emotional level, it is antidepressant, calming, and uplifting. It has similarities both to neroli and bergamot.
OTHER USES: Flatulence, nausea and vomiting; as an insect repellant.

Rosewood
Aniba rosaeodora
Though this oil is actually extracted from the tropical evergreen rosewood tree, it has the relaxing and emotional balancing qualities associated with the more expensive essence of rose and is often used as a substitute for it. It has a sweet, floral fragrance, though not the heady quality of rose, and blends well with sandalwood, bergamot, and geranium. It has a calming, steadying effect and is good for insomnia, headaches, nervous tension, and nausea. It also stimulates the immune system.
OTHER USES: General skin care; colds, coughs and flu.

Orange *(below)*
(Citrus sinensis)
This third of the orange oils comes from the rind of the fruit and has a soothing and uplifting quality and a sweet, fresh smell. It is a relaxing essence and is helpful in stress-related conditions and insomnia. It blends well with spicy oils such as clove, or with lavender and clary sage. *Like most citrus oils, it should not be used on the skin before exposure to sunlight.*
OTHER USES: Colds, flu and bronchitis; water retention; skin care for oily skin.

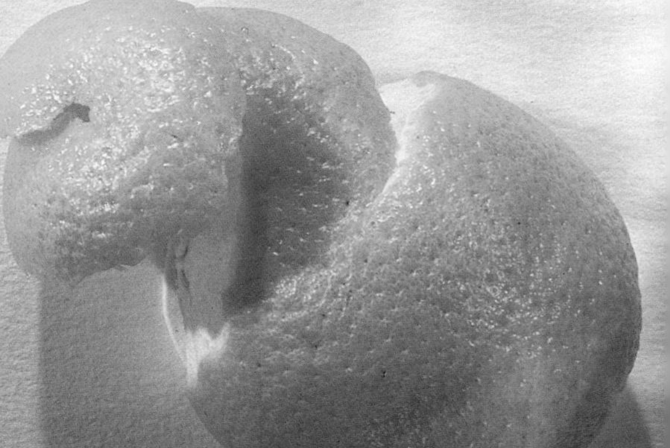

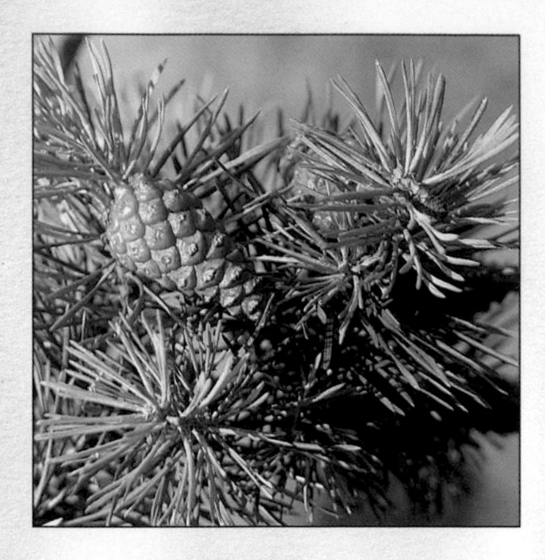

Pine *(above)*
(Pinus sylvestris)
This refreshing, stimulating oil has a clean smell of pine and makes an excellent inhalant for blocked sinuses, catarrh, and general congestion. It is also used for rheumatism, arthritis, and muscular aches and pains where it has a quite invigorating effect. It works on an emotional level in much the same way as cypress and is good for nervous exhaustion and fatigue. Also, like cypress, it is a natural deodorant. Blend with cedarwood, rosemary, and patchouli.
Other uses: Cystitis and urinary infections.

Camphor
(Cinnamomum camphora)
Camphor oil is extracted from the wood of this tropical evergreen tree. As an essential oil, it can have a very marked effect when used by a trained aromatherapist. However, as it can be a strong stimulant to the heart, it is best left to the professional therapists and only for severe ailments. In this context, however, it has various uses – respiratory ailments, for both diarrhea and constipation, and as a tonic for the heart, the circulation of the blood, and the respiratory system.

Black pepper *(below)*
(Piper nigrum)
Essence of black pepper has a warm, spicy scent and a stimulating, warming action both physically and emotionally. It is a good remedy for colds, flu, and fever. It also acts on the digestive system, on colic, constipation, diarrhea, flatulence, and loss of appetite. It stimulates the circulation and is helpful before and after exercise, as it warms up the muscles and is good for sprains. It should only be used very moderately, mixed with other essences such as frankincense, sandalwood, lavender, and rosemary.
Other uses: Rheumatism and arthritis; anemia; hemorrhoids.

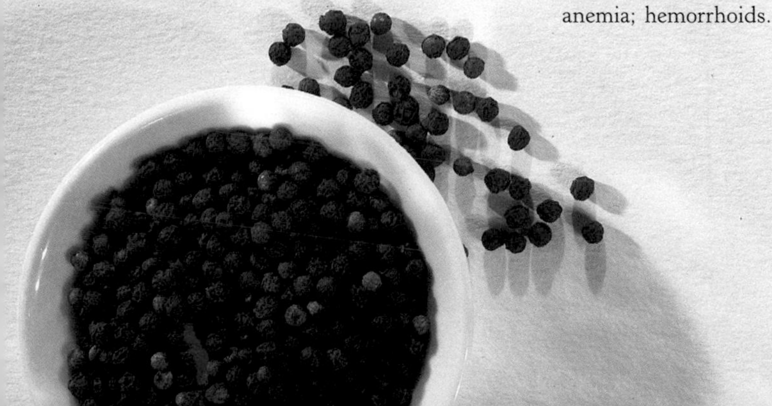

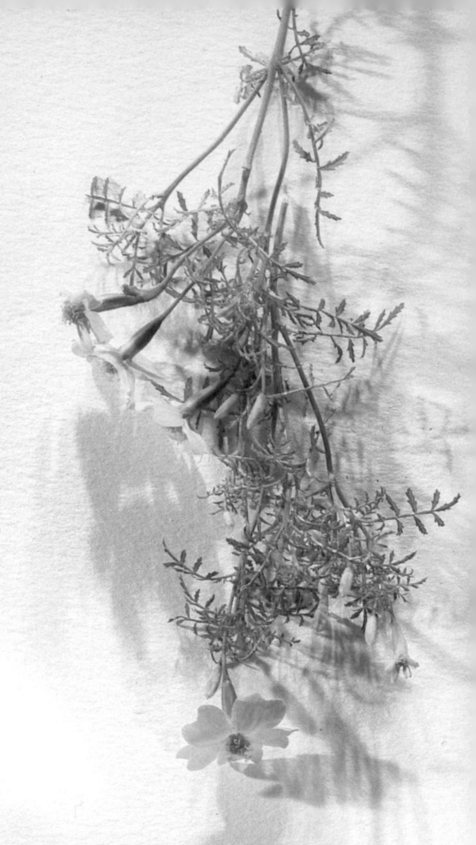

Tagetes *(above)*
(Tagetes minuta)
Although this oil comes from a plant closely related to French and African marigolds, it is often wrongly confused with the true marigold, the oil from which is rarely available. It is an excellent air freshener and insect repellant. Inhaled in this way, it promotes mental stimulation. It blends well with clary sage, lavender, and bergamot, *but it should be used extremely sparingly on the skin.*
Other uses: Bunions, callouses, and corns.

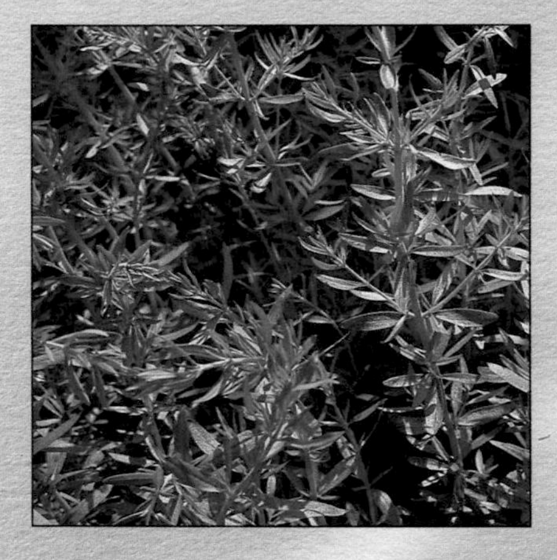

Patchouli
(Pogostemon patchouli)
The strong sensual odor of patchouli will forever be associated with the hippy 1960s! It is renowned as an anti-depressant and aphrodisiac, and is one of the few oils to improve with age. It is useful on cracked or chapped skin and in cases of acne, athlete's foot, and eczema. It blends well with lavender, sandalwood, myrrh, neroli, and clary sage.
OTHER USES: For oily skin and hair; for sharpening and focusing the mind.

Cardamon *(below)*
(Elettaria cardamomum)
Although this is a warming, sweet, slightly gingery essence, it shares many properties with peppermint. They combine well together and are excellent for nausea and heartburn. It is good for use in the bath and has an uplifting, calming – and, some say, aphrodisiac – effect on the emotions.
OTHER USES: As a general tonic, especially for those with nervous problems.

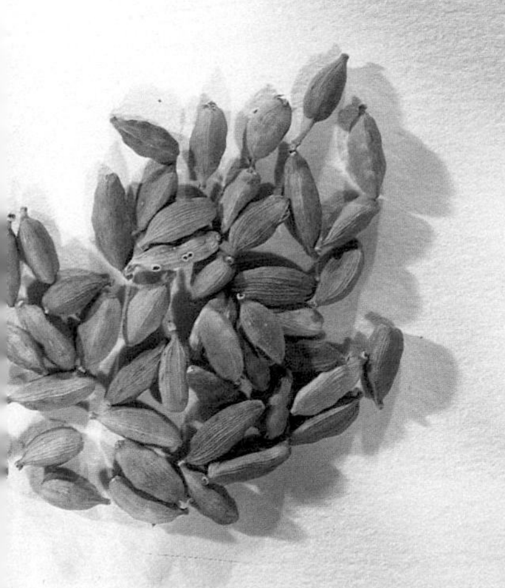

Hyssop *(above)*
(Hyssopus officinalis)
The essential oil that comes from the hyssop herb has a wide variety of uses. However, it should not be used by people who suffer from epilepsy or during pregnancy, and as it does seem to have a somewhat toxic effect, it is best left to the use of a professional aromatherapist. Having said this, it is an excellent tonic when used properly – especially for people convalescing after a long illness.
OTHER USES: For bronchitis, asthma and catarrh, on bruises and wounds.

Citronella
(Cymbopogon nardus)
This powerful lemon-scented oil comes from a grass found in Sri Lanka. It is often used on a vaporizer to scent a room or to repel insects. It is used in skin care for oily skin and as a deodorant. It has a clear, uplifting quality and so is good for nervous exhaustion, headaches, and migraine. Use only in small quantities and blend with geranium, bergamot, cedarwood, and pine.
OTHER USES: As an antiseptic; for minor infections.

Grapefruit *(below)*
(Citrus paradisi)
This uplifting, refreshing oil has much in common with other citrus essences, and it blends well with these herbal and spicy oils. It is a good toner for oily hair and skin, and it also lifts the spirits, making it effective against depression, exhaustion, and nervous stress. It makes a good oil for an early morning bath before a busy day. However, use it soon after purchase as it loses its power more quickly than most oils.
OTHER USES: Cellulite and water retention; colds and flu.

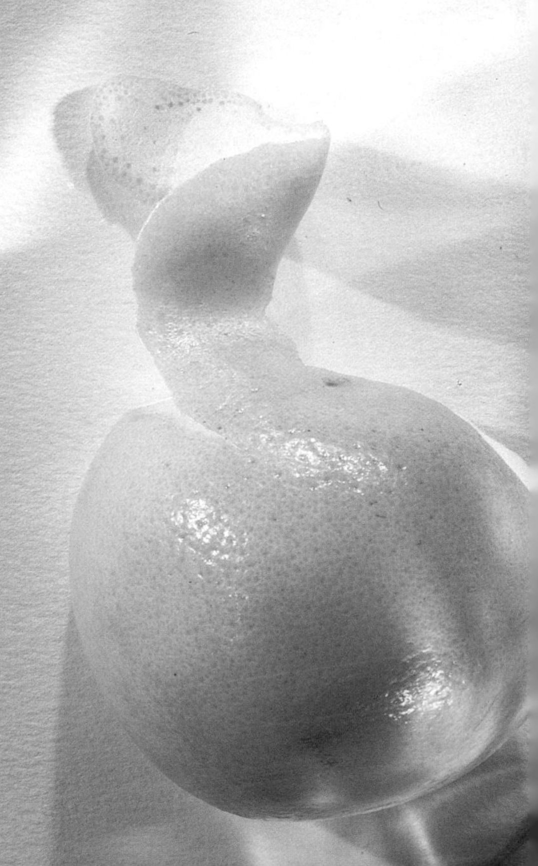

BASIC TECHNIQUES

Essential oils work on the body in two principal ways: absorption through the skin and inhalation through the olfactory system (see page 6). A wide variety of methods of using the oils has therefore evolved, from steam inhalations to massage. Some methods are best suited to particular conditions; for instance, a steam inhalation with eucalyptus oil is ideal for congestion caused by a cold. Pressure of time and circumstances are other considerations – a massage may be impossible during the working day, but breathing in basil oil from a tissue can give your concentration and mental energy an instant boost.

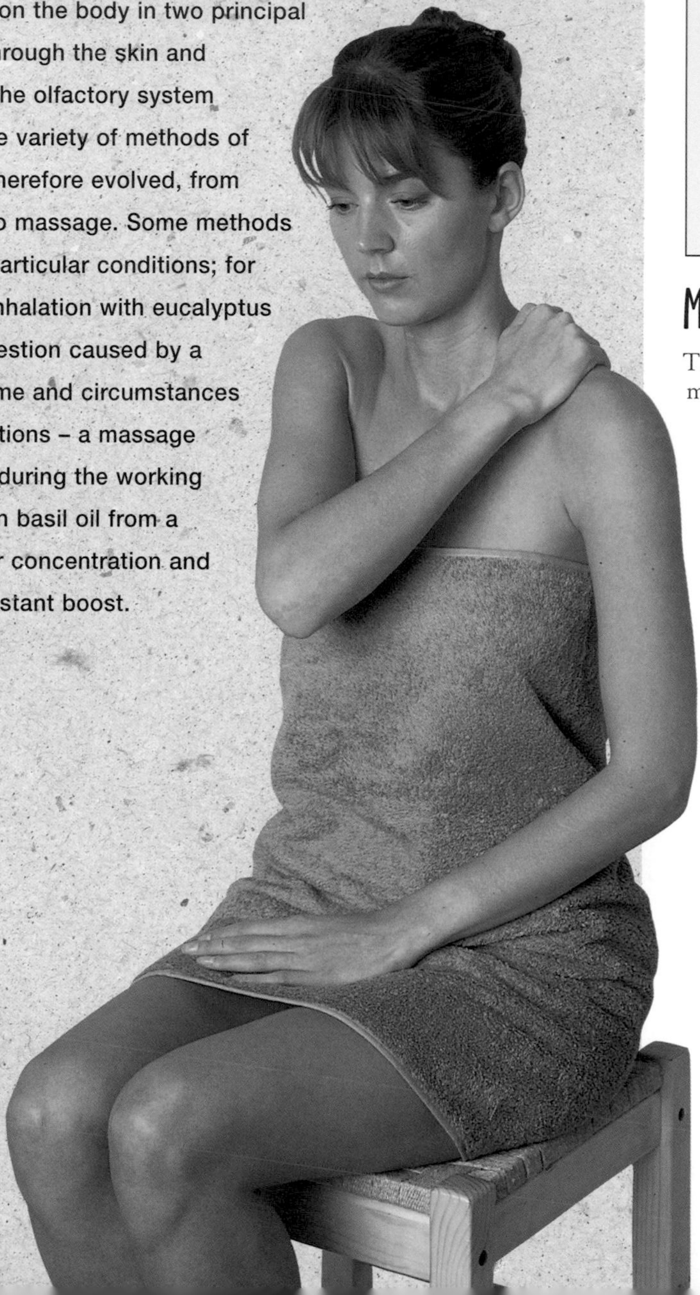

While a full body massage is a real treat and the ultimate in relaxation, you can use spot do-it-yourself massage for areas of tension.

WARNING

As a general rule, essential oils are applied to the skin only when diluted in a carrier oil. There are a few cases, however, where pure oil is used – for instance, lavender on burns, cuts, and insect stings. Most oils should not be used in this way, and as the results can be quite painful, don't be tempted to experiment!

MASSAGE

This is probably the best known method of using aromatherapy oils. The effect of a good massage is wonderful, as the oils penetrate through the olfactory system as well as the skin, and there are the important benefits of the massage itself. The oils are always blended in a carrier oil (see page 22), and the mixture will depend upon any particular condition that is being addressed as well as personal preference.

A full body massage is demonstrated on pages 24-37, and there are individual self-help massage techniques given in the Specific Applications section (pages 38-59).

COMPRESSES

Compresses have two main uses: to reduce swellings and sprains, and to soothe headaches. Use a clean piece of cotton fabric (a handkerchief or a towel, depending on the area to be covered). Add the essential oil to the water (1–8 drops depending on how large the compress is) and mix well. Soak the fabric, squeeze it out, and place over the affected area. Use warm water for muscular aches, ice-cold water for headaches and sprains.

As the compress cools down or heats up, re-soak and re-apply. The longer you leave the compress on, the better, preferably at least an hour.

BATHS

Some oil in the bathwater before bedtime if you suffer from insomnia can give a good night's rest (lavender is particularly good). Baths are also useful for conditions such as rheumatism and arthritis where there is painful swelling making massage inappropriate. Add 5–10 drops of oil to the water when you have filled the tub. It should not be too hot, as this would make the oil evaporate. Swish the water to mix in the oil before you get in. Sitz or hip baths (or a plastic bowl) are useful for vaginal disorders and genitourinary infections.

STEAM INHALATIONS

Pour boiling water into a bowl, add 10 drops of the appropriate oil and breathe in deeply, covering your head and the bowl with a towel. Stay for about 10 minutes. This is very good for sinus, throat, and chest infections, but *this method is not to be used if you have asthma.*

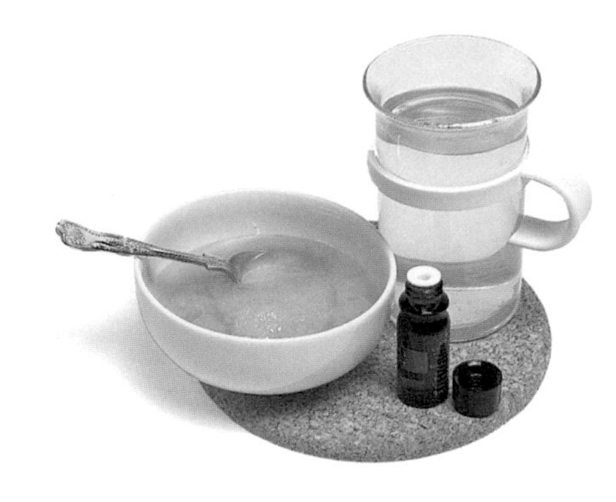

Occasionally, the essential oils may be taken internally in hot water, with a teaspoonful of honey added.

ON PILLOWS AND TISSUES

This is perhaps the simplest use of essential oils, but nonetheless very effective. A drop of lavender or rose oil on the pillow at night gives a deep, restful sleep. A drop of peppermint oil on a tissue can relieve a headache, while oils such as jasmine and clary sage inhaled from a tissue can boost low spirits.

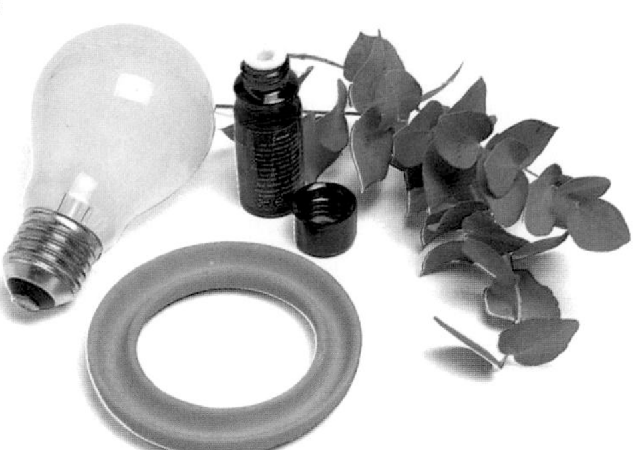

A few drops of oil on a burner or light bulb ring will scent an entire room.

HONEY WATER

In the rare cases where internal use is recommended, honey water is preferable to plain. Put a teaspoonful of honey in a cup of hot water and stir until dissolved. Then add a drop of the appropriate oil – *but only those specifically suggested in this book.* Use honey water, too, as a base for mouthwashes and gargles.

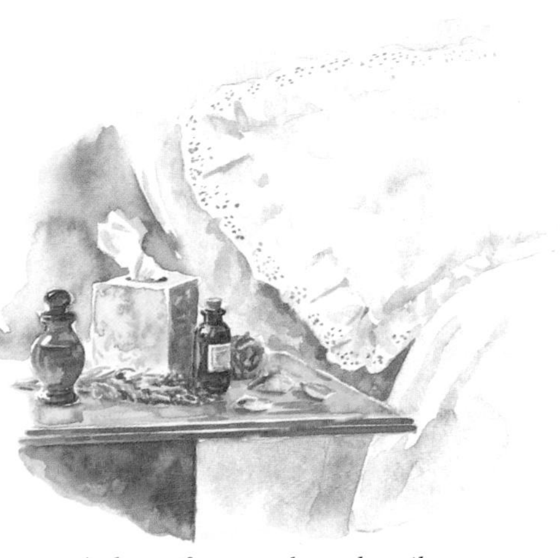

A drop of rose or lavender oil on your pillow will guarantee a good night's sleep.

VAPORIZATION

You can buy special aromatherapy oil burners or light bulb rings to which you add a few drops of essential oil – your choice of oil depends on whether you require antibacterial properties (rosemary and eucalyptus are ideal) or you just want to give a pleasant scent to a room. You can also put a few drops of oil directly onto a radiator or in a bowl of warm water to achieve the same effect.

Using the Oils

Essential oils are extremely volatile – they will evaporate rapidly or deteriorate if kept in the wrong conditions. Only buy oils that are sold in airtight, dark glass bottles (never plastic). Do not expose them unstoppered to the air or to sunlight and keep them in a cool, dry place, preferably a refrigerator (though NEVER a freezer).

Carrier Oils

As a general rule, aromatherapy oils must be diluted in a carrier oil before they can be applied to the skin. Various types of oil can be used, and any cold-pressed vegetable oil will make a good base. One consideration is the smell – olive oil, for instance, has quite an overpowering smell. Almond, grapeseed, peach, or apricot kernel oils are vitamin-rich and easily absorbed. Olive and wheatgerm oils are usually used with another lighter carrier oil and are particularly good for dry and mature skin, and for a massage oil to be used on the face. Coconut oil blends well with sweet floral essences. Calendula oil is excellent for problem skin.

If you want to make up a quantity of massage oil for future use, bear in mind that both vegetable and essential oils oxidize and become rancid. Keeping them, once mixed, in dark glass airtight bottles is essential. Wheatgerm oil prevents oxidization, so always use a little of this (10% or more) as part of your carrier oil.

Dark glass bottles in various sizes are usually available from pharmacies for storing your blended oils.

Recommended Dilutions

FOR USE ON THE BODY	FOR USE ON CHILDREN
25 drops of essential oil in *2 oz. (50ml) carrier oil*	*10 drops of essential oil* in *2 oz. (50ml) carrier oil*
FOR USE ON THE FACE	**FOR USE ON BABIES**
12 drops of essential oil in *2 oz. (50ml) carrier oil*	*5 drops of essential oil* in *2 oz. (50ml) carrier oil*

Essential oils are always diluted in carrier oils (see the table above). Peach, apricot, grapeseed, almond, coconut, calendula, olive, and wheatgerm oil are all recommended.

Blending Essential Oils

Blending essential oils is often made – rather unnecessarily – into something of a mystery. It is, in fact, a combination of common sense and personal preference. Start by measuring the correct amount of carrier oil into a dark glass bottle. If you are following one of the recipes in this book, measure in the number of drops given for each essence, stopper, shake the bottle well, and, if you are not going to use it all immediately, label it.

If, however, you decide to experiment with blending, follow the simple maxim: you can add but you cannot take away. So add drops very gradually, mix and see if you feel that the blend is going to be what you want. Three (or occasionally four) should be the maximum number of essences used in any mixture. If you use more than this, the overall aroma can become muddied.

Interestingly, it is very common that the oils you like the smell of are the very ones you need therapeutically – so this is one time when you can certainly be led by your nose.

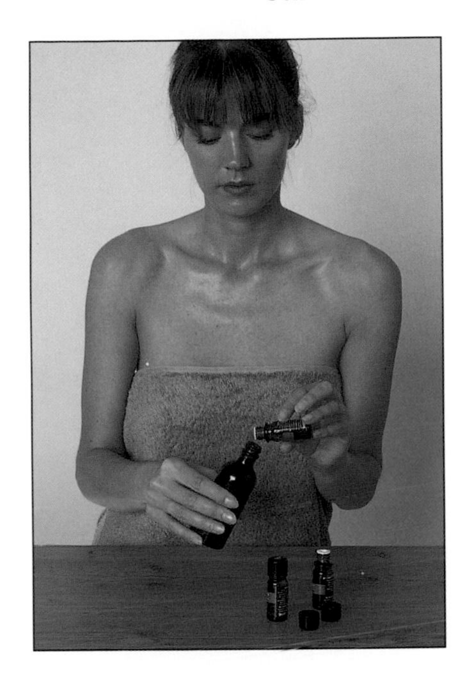

Aromatherapy oils should always be kept in dark glass bottles to protect them from the light. Put the carrier oil in first and add essential oils gradually until you achieve a scent you like.

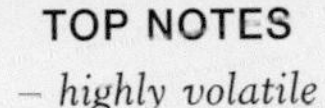

In perfumery, oils are divided into groups of *top notes* (highly volatile, such as the citrus oils); *middle notes* (less volatile, such as clary sage and neroli); and *bass notes* (the longest-lasting, which give stability to the blend, such as sandalwood). A classic blend, using this method would take one from each of the groups of notes to give a balanced effect. It is not necessary, however, to follow this pattern, and there are many arguments about in which groups the various oils belong! Another approach to blending is to stick to a family of essences – for instance, using oils that all come from herbs or all from citrus fruits. In fact, there are few hard and fast rules when it comes to blending, and you will find, with familiarity, you will start instinctively to put particular oils together.

TOP NOTES

– highly volatile

Examples include: Citrus oils, such as grapefruit, lemon, and orange

MIDDLE NOTES

– less volatile

Examples include: Clary sage and neroli

BOTTOM NOTES

– most stable

Examples include: Sandalwood

MASSAGE BASICS

Massage is one of the most ancient healing arts. It is also an instinctive response to pain – a mother will automatically "rub it better" if her child falls over. In aromatherapy terms, massage is used to help the skin to absorb the oils, as well as to encourage the body to relax. Besides relaxing tense muscles, massage can help to eliminate toxins via the skin, stimulate the circulation, and, most importantly, ease mental and emotional tensions.

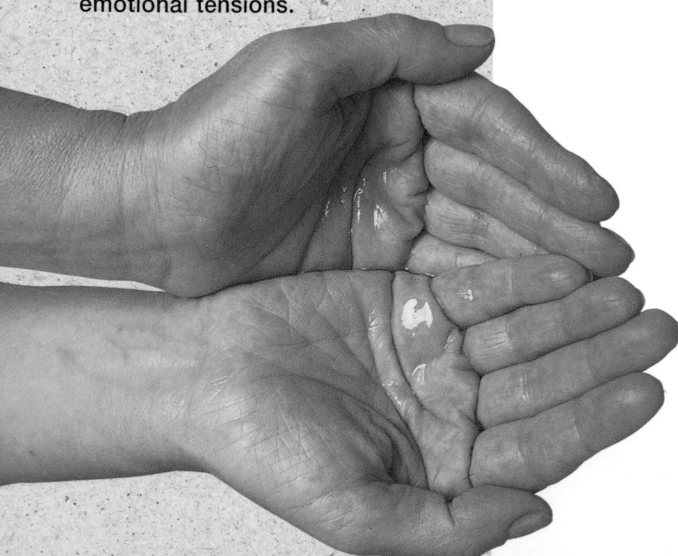

Always take time to warm the oil in your hands before the massage – the last thing your partner wants is the shock of cold oil!

As the overall aim of aromatherapy massage is relaxation, the basic strokes used are gentle. The more vigorous of the strokes used in conventional Swedish massage are inappropriate. There are various methods of self-massage mentioned in the Specific Applications section of this book (pages 38-59). Here, though, the focus is on how to do a full massage. Obviously, for this, you will need a partner who will reciprocate in massaging you, too, and in this way, you will both benefit from this most luxurious and relaxing of treatments.

It is important to trust your instincts when giving a massage. Rely on your sense of touch. You will feel knotted-up muscles that need to be released, and these areas may require more concentrated work. However, go gently. If you go too deeply or vigorously into an already tense muscle, it may react by going into a spasm of greater tension. Always ask if the pressure is too strong or not strong enough. Gradually, as you become more familiar with and confident of your sense of touch, you will find your hands seeming to know instinctively exactly what is needed.

Cold muscles do not relax, so it is important to keep those parts of the body that are not being worked on covered up with towels. As a rough guide, one towel is needed to lie on and at least two more to use as covers. Always work in a warm room. Ideally, you should use a massage table, but it is unlikely you will have access to one. You can use the floor (if you don't have a bad back – bending over can put a strain on it) or a bed.

CONTRA-INDICATIONS

There are a number of conditions when you should NOT give a massage:

Pain or inflammation of any kind is a warning sign, and you should not give a massage over these areas – for instance:

- Joints swollen by rheumatism or arthritis.
- Broken, infectious, or septic skin or recent scar tissue must be avoided.
- If there is any unusual lump or bump, do not touch it.
- Varicose veins should never be massaged.
- Do not massage anyone with a heart condition.
- Do not massage breasts or glandular tissue.

PREPARATION FOR MASSAGE

When you give a massage, you need to concentrate on it fully. So make sure you are not going to be disturbed. Choose a time – allowing yourself at least an hour and a half – when you are not going to have visitors and switch on the answering machine or unplug the phone.

The room should be warmer than you would usually have it and the lighting should be subdued. Wear loose, comfortable clothes that you can move freely in and no jewelry. You can either work in silence or play soothing music very quietly in the background.

It is best to be completely naked when being massaged – the areas not being worked on should be covered up with towels. If you are giving the massage, settle your partner under the towels and take a moment to concentrate your energies. For the next hour or so, try to leave everything else behind and live just through your sense of touch. Don't talk to your partner – unless it is to ask about the massage itself – and let any communication take place on the level of touch.

Let your whole body move in rhythm with the strokes – it is much easier than merely using the strength in your arms. Finally, always warm the oil in the palms of your hands before you apply it – applied cold, it would be a shock to your partner.

AFTER THE MASSAGE

Give your partner time to resurface – don't suddenly turn up the lights or make a noise. Wash your hands and arms in cold water to eliminate any negativity picked up from your partner during the massage. The oils will continue to work after the massage itself has finished, so don't be tempted to rush to the shower to wash it all off. The best time to receive a massage is in the evening so you can go to bed and let the oils work on your skin through the night.

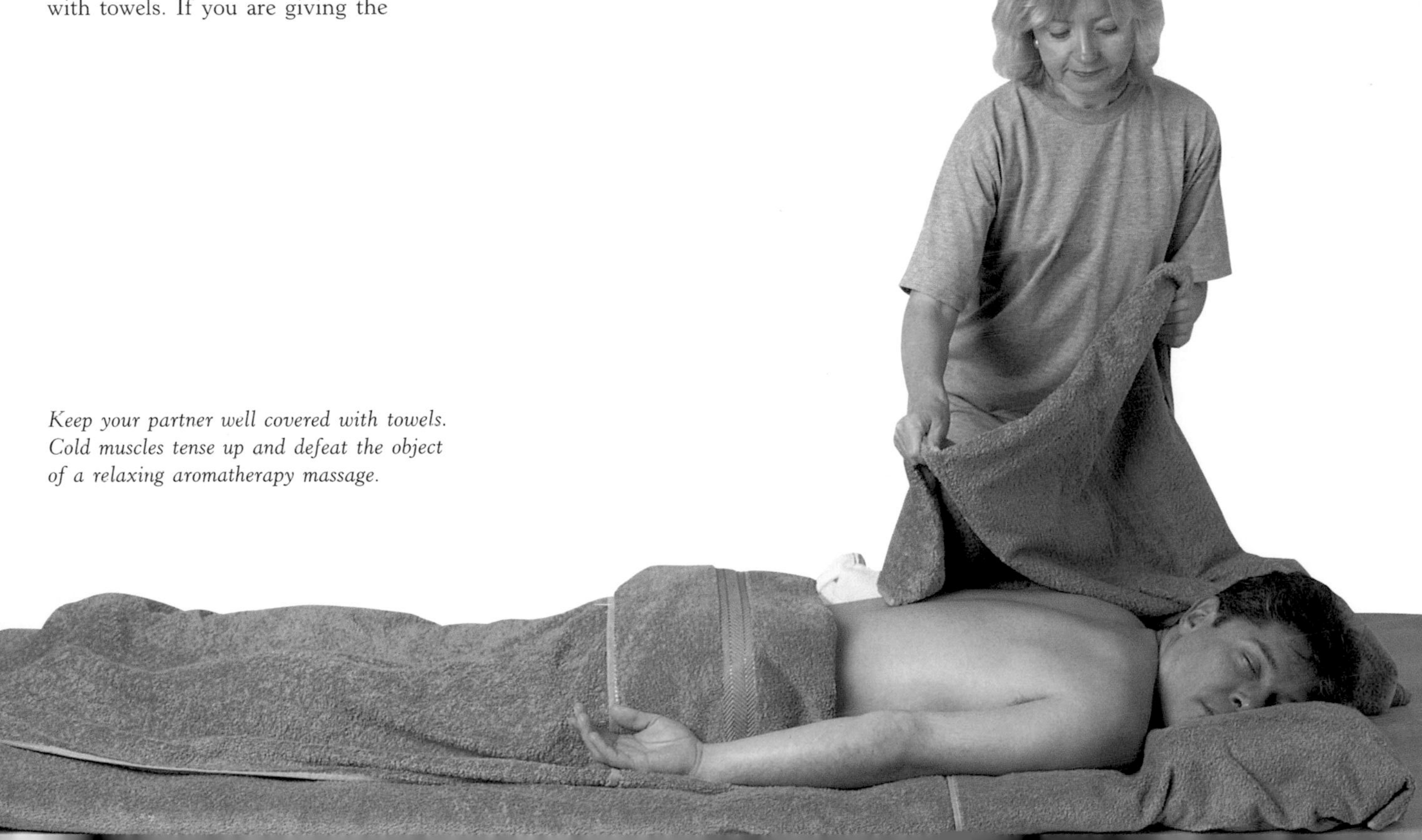

Keep your partner well covered with towels. Cold muscles tense up and defeat the object of a relaxing aromatherapy massage.

The Basic Massage Strokes

Aromatherapy massage has the ultimate aim of relaxation – so there is little of the vigorous hacking used in conventional massage – though it does have a small part to play, and the technique is demonstrated here.

Although this full body massage follows a set pattern of strokes, it is important to remember that instinct and intuition have a vital part to play. If a particular stroke has a marked effect, you will no doubt want to repeat it. Conversely, if anything hurts, stop. Allow your hands to feel their own way and be your guide. The strokes mentioned here are only the basics. Once you have mastered them, you can find out more from a good massage book or simply by trying things out yourself.

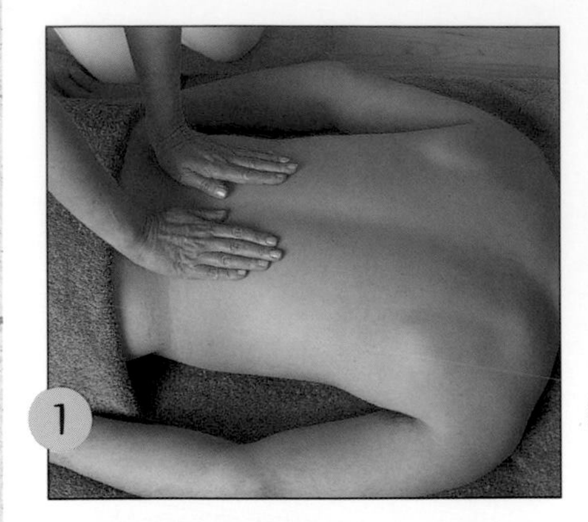

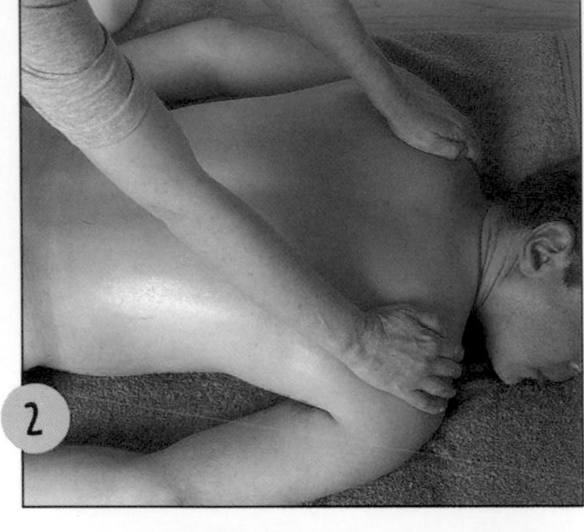

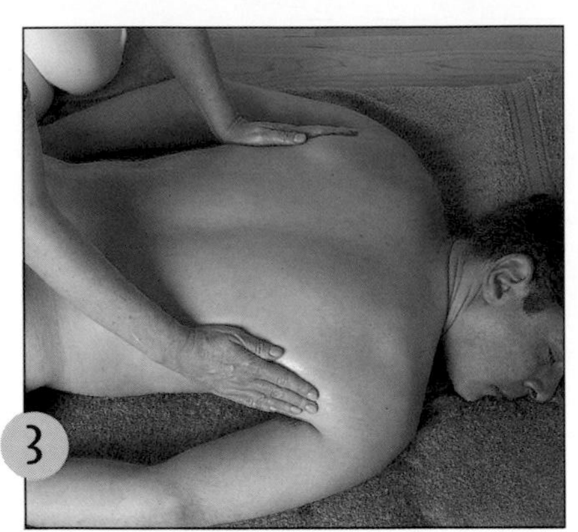

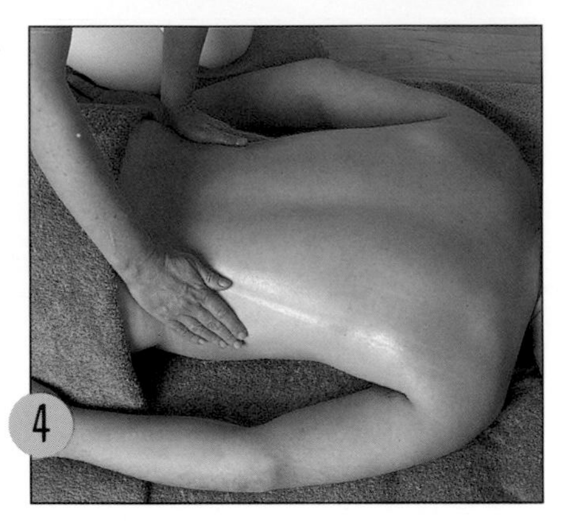

Effleurage

Effleurage is a long, slow rhythmic movement sometimes described as stroking, and it is the most important of the techniques used in aromatherapy massage. It is done with the flat of the hands, with the fingers closed together and pointing upward, as far as possible as you move.

There should be a firm, even pressure as the hands move toward the heart, and a lighter, more gliding touch on their return. Effleurage is used at the beginning and end of each stage of the massage.

At the start, it spreads oil over the body and establishes nonverbal contact with your partner. At the end, it is a signal that you have finished working on that area. From this point on, each repetition of the movement becomes lighter and lighter with every stroke, ending with a feather-like touch.

When massaging the back, in particular, it is a good idea to end the effleurage with the stroke known as feather stroke (see page 33).

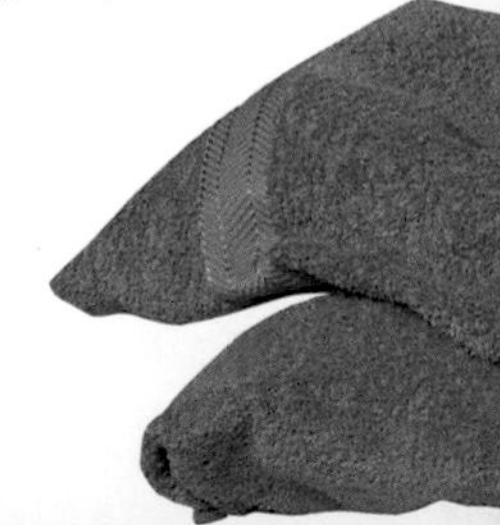

PETRISSAGE

Petrissage uses the fingers or thumbs to squeeze soft tissue against the bone immediately beneath it. It helps to eliminate accumulated toxins.

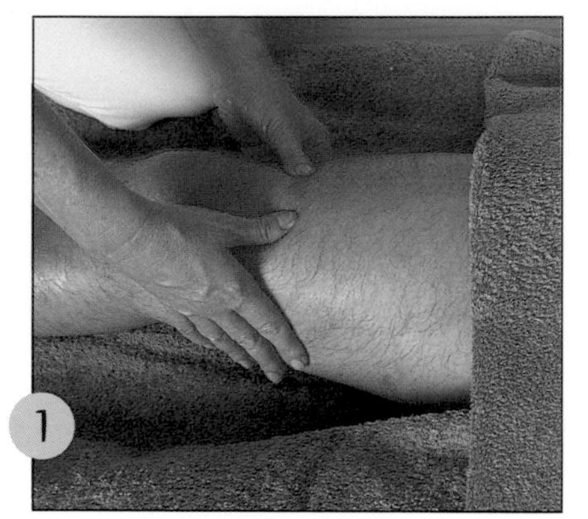

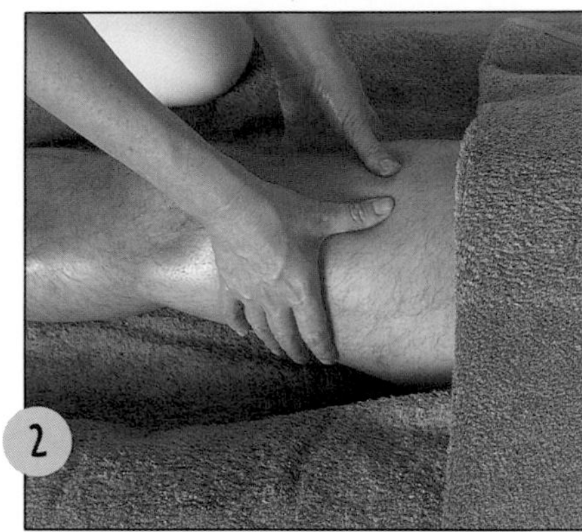

KNEADING

Kneading – the movement is just like kneading bread – is applied to soft tissue that has no bone immediately beneath it. You pick up the flesh and roll it away from the bone with a squeezing action. It relaxes tense muscles, stimulates the circulation, and eliminates toxins.

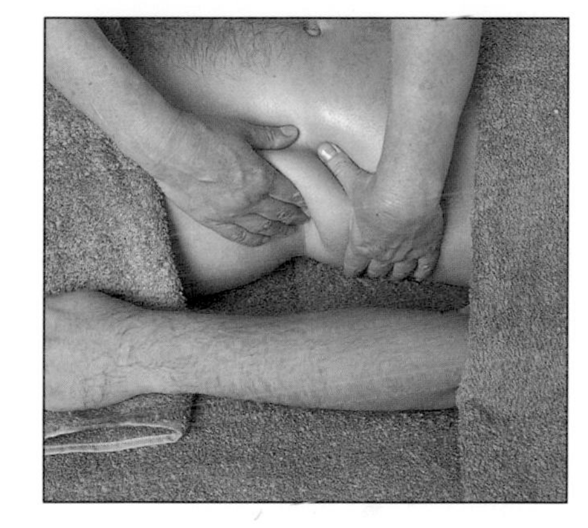

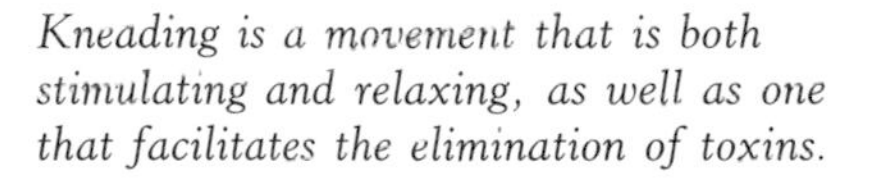

Kneading is a movement that is both stimulating and relaxing, as well as one that facilitates the elimination of toxins.

CUPPING

This is another quick movement. The hands form the shape of a cup and make a vacuum where they meet the skin. The resulting sound is like a horse trotting. Quick, alternating strokes make this an excellent toner for the circulation.

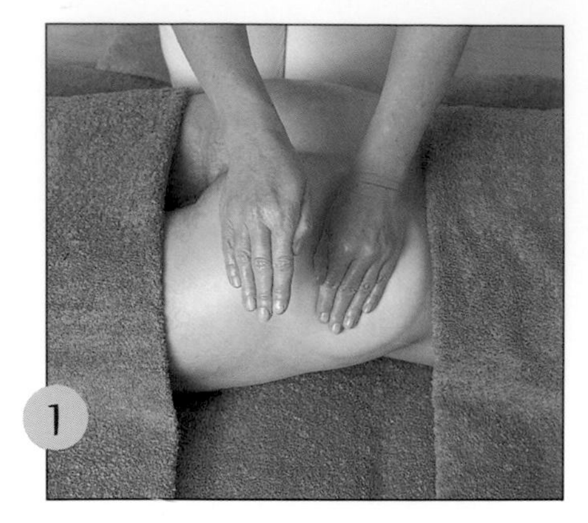

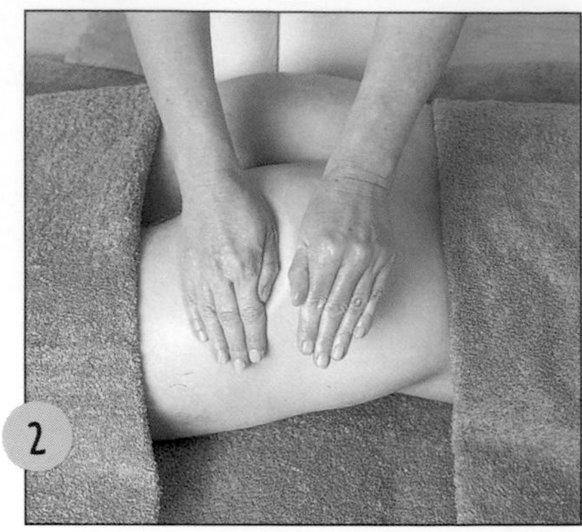

HACKING

This is a stimulating movement and only to be used very lightly and gently in aromatherapy massage. It is done using the outside edge of the little fingers, alternating in a chopping movement on areas like the calves, thighs, and buttocks. Keep the hands very loose, or it will be too sharp an action. This stroke is not used if the massage is aiming to induce deep relaxation.

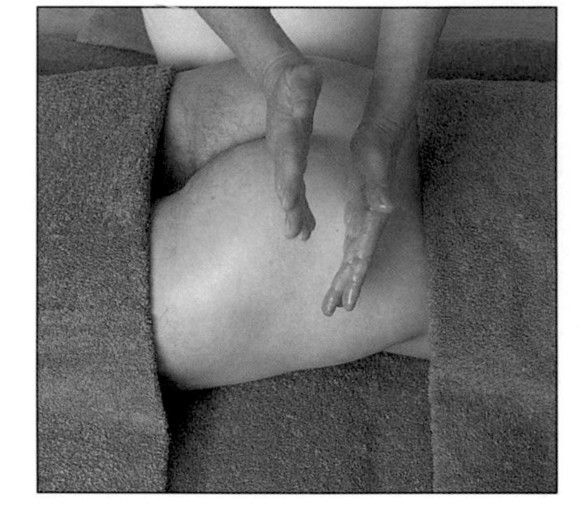

Hacking is a relatively strong movement for aromatherapy massage and only used on less sensitive areas like the calves, thighs, and buttocks.

Full Body Massage

Start the massage with your partner lying face down. Make sure he or she is warm and comfortable, and covered completely with two towels, one across the top of the body and the other over the buttocks and legs. Begin by asking your partner to take some slow, deep breaths as this will help promote relaxation. It is a good idea to do this deep breathing together as it will relax you, too, and make you feel centered.

Before you begin, make sure you are not going to be disturbed. Take the phone off the hook or switch on the answer machine.

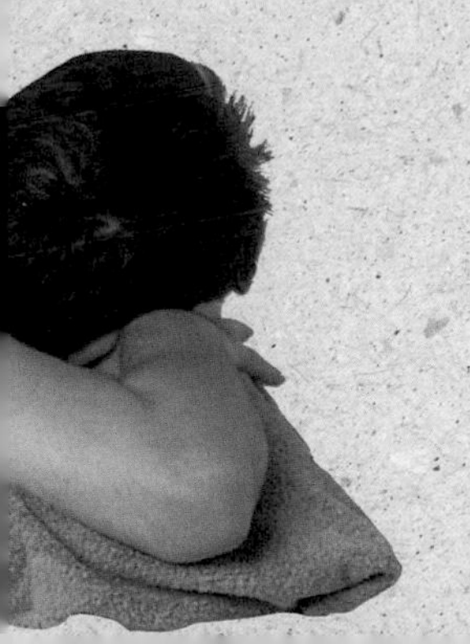

Legs

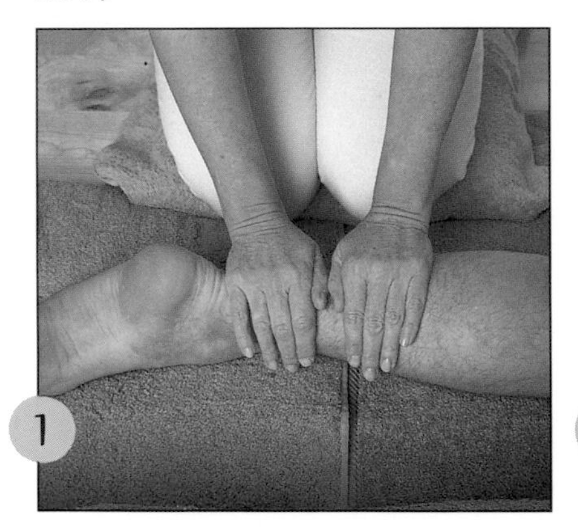

1

Uncover the right leg.

Warm some massage oil in the palms of your hands and place them flat next to each other at the bottom of the leg, near the ankle.

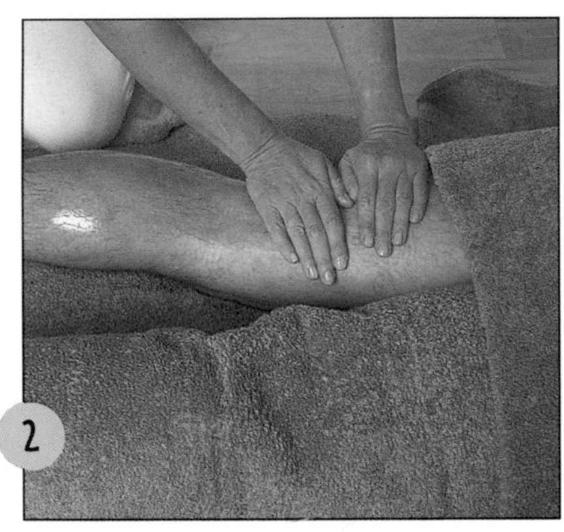

2

Gently but firmly effleurage up the center of the leg, keeping your hands close together and your fingers closed.

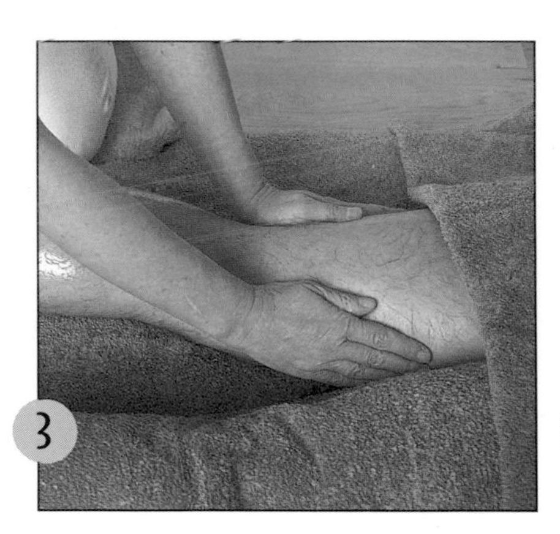

3

At the top of the leg, turn your hands so your fingers are facing up and move them to the outside of the thigh.

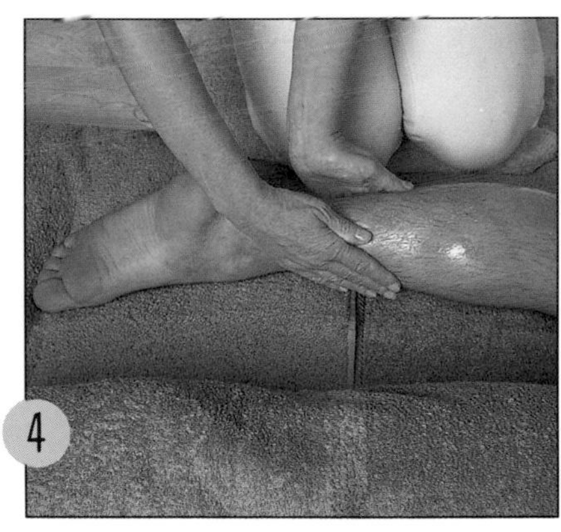

4

In a long, even sweep, bring your hands down the outer sides of the leg to the ankle. In a seamless movement, turn them so they are ready to go up the leg again. Repeat several times.

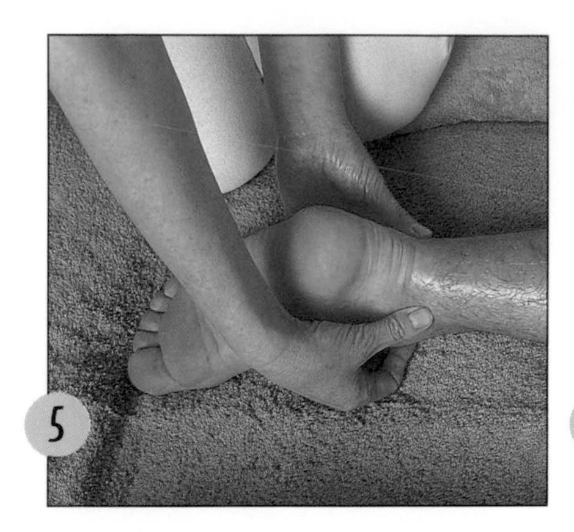

Petrissage to each side of the ankle around the ankle bone. Do not press on the bone itself.

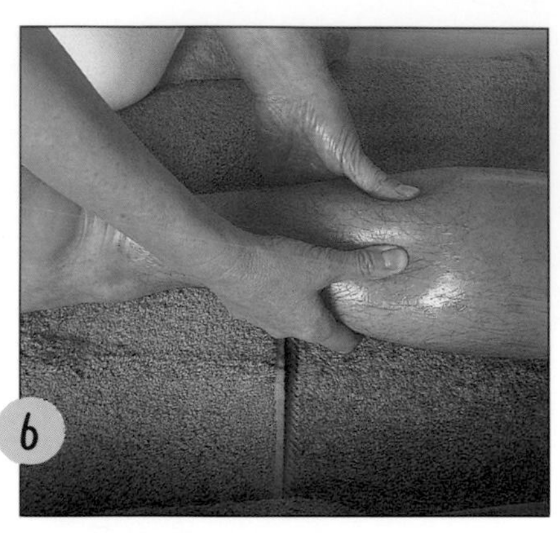

Continue the movement all the way up the center of the leg. Be sensitive – petrissage may be too deep for some areas, particularly the back of the knee.

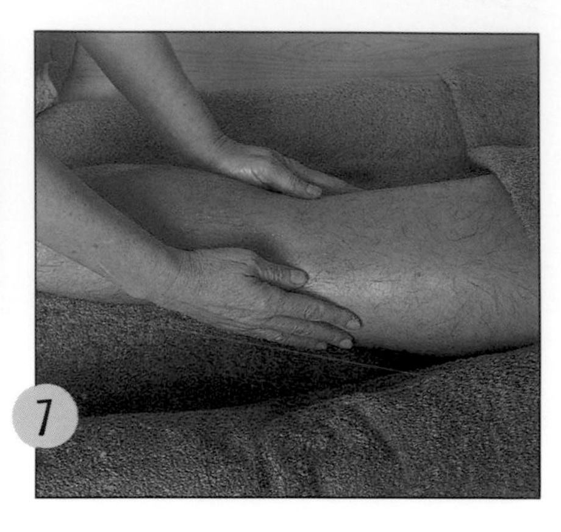

At the top of the thigh, take your hands to the outside of the leg and bring them back down to the ankle in one long sweeping movement. Repeat this several times.

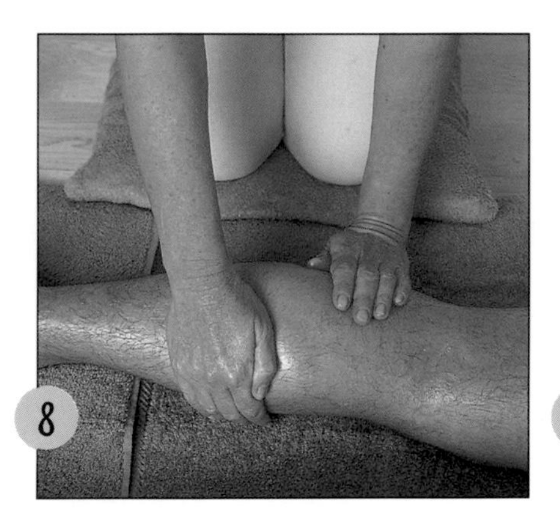

This movement – alternate effleurage – is quite vigorous and stimulating. Start at the ankle, with your hands together, and then take them in opposite directions, alternating as you go.

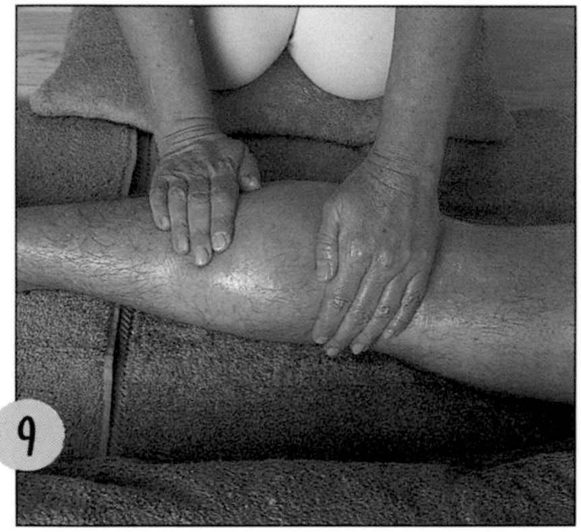

Alternate effleurage from the ankle to the top of the thigh, using the gentler stroking movement down the outer leg, as before, to return to the ankle. Repeat several times.

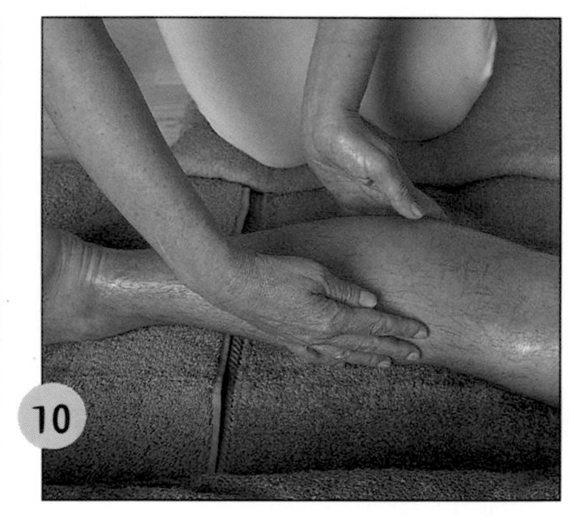

Effleurage, as at the beginning, several times, getting lighter each time. Cover the leg and repeat on the left leg.

BUTTOCKS

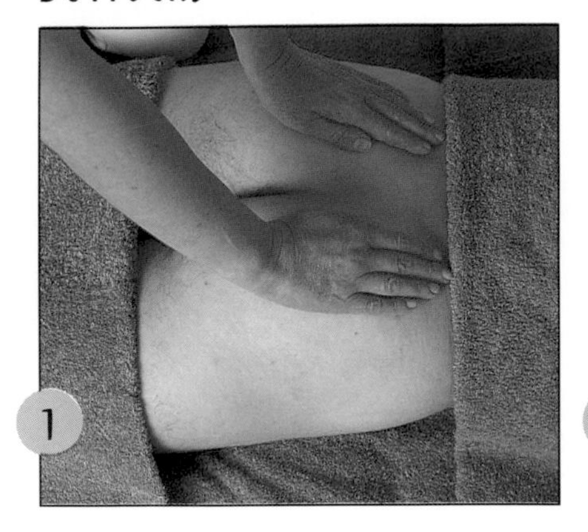

1

Put some more oil in your palms and warm it. Uncover the buttocks and lay one hand on each cheek.

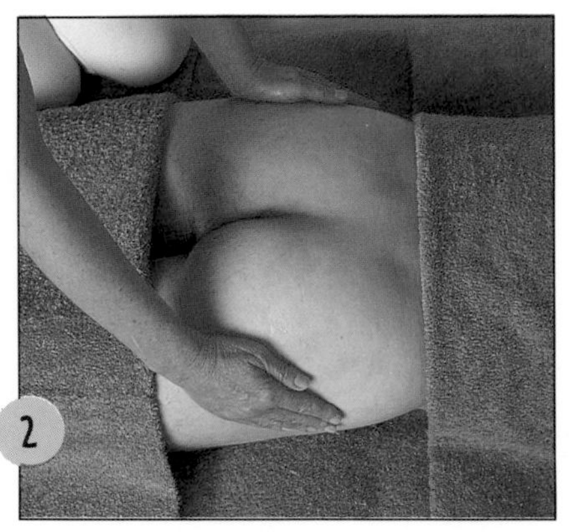

2

Effleurage with firm circular movements, spreading the oil over the whole area as you go.

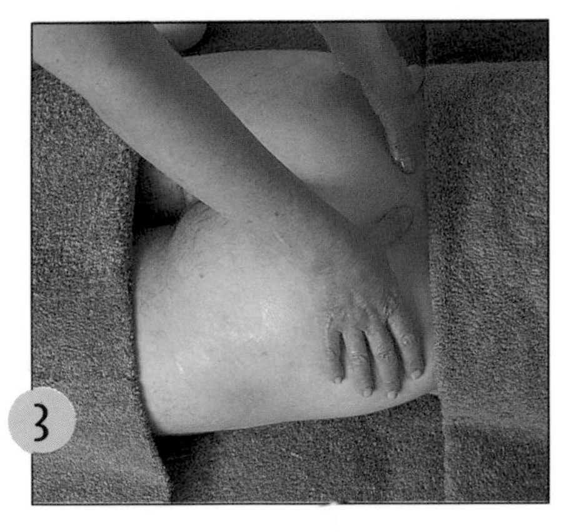

3

Petrissage both cheeks, starting at the spine and working out toward the sides with a deep pressure.

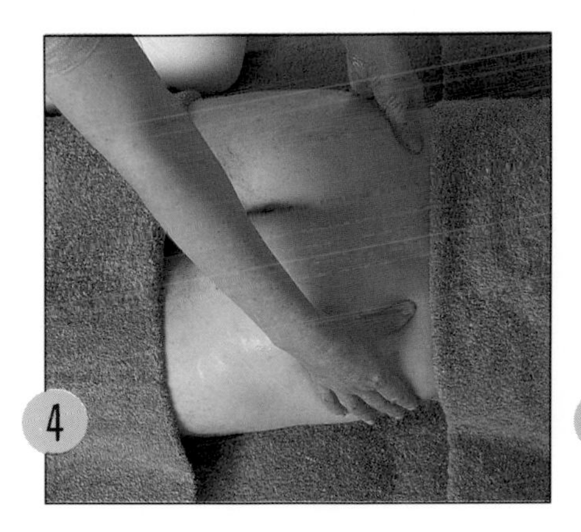

4

Work across the whole surface, moving down an inch each time until you reach the base of the spine. Always remember to start about an inch out from the spine – never work on the spine itself.

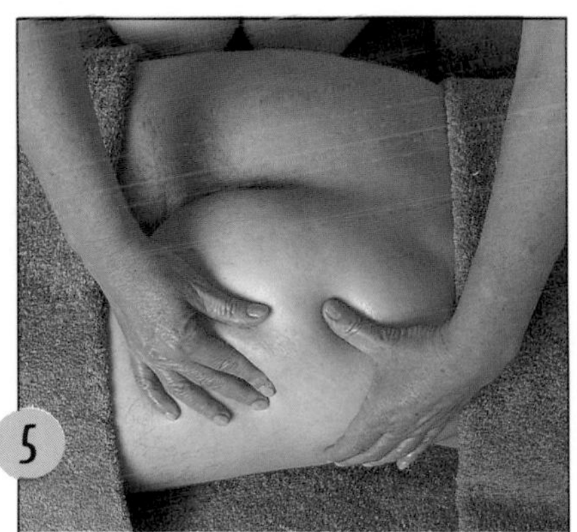

5

From one side of the body knead the opposite cheek. Then change sides and knead the other side.

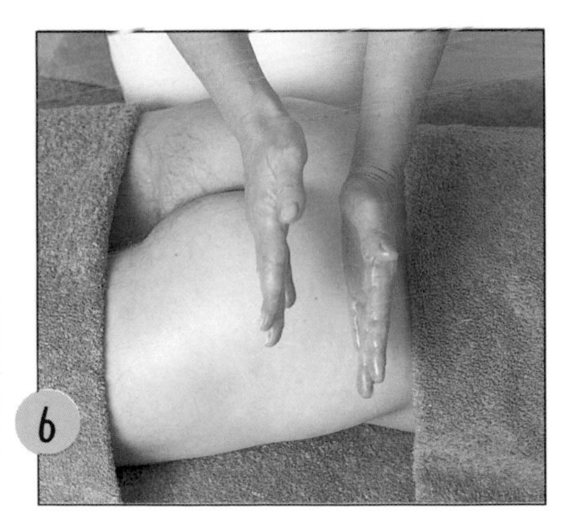

6

Hack and cup (see page 28) the whole cheek, then effleurage. Swap sides and repeat. Effleurage as at the start, with lighter and lighter pressure. Cover the buttocks and uncover the back.

BACK

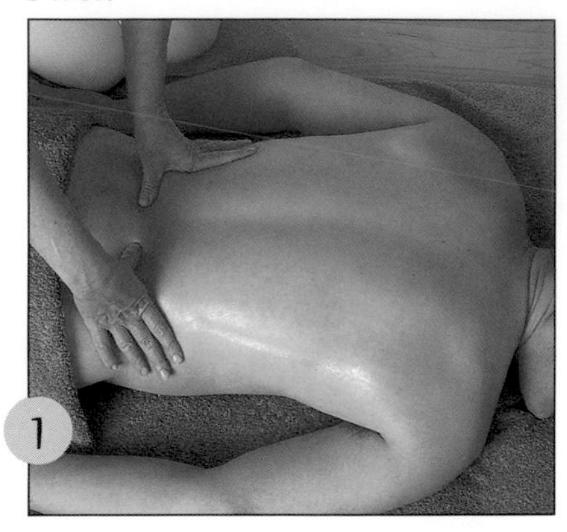

Place your hands at the base of the spine and effleurage up to the neck, gliding out over the shoulders and returning down the sides (see page 26). Repeat several times. Move your hands back to the base of the spine.

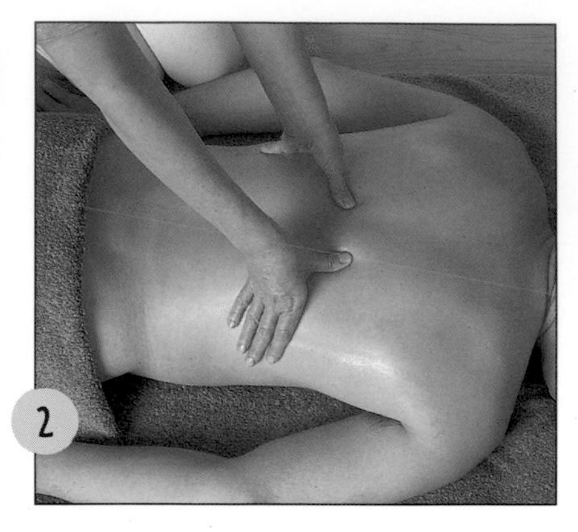

With a circular movement of your thumbs, petrissage up from the base of the spine to the neck, working next to the spine, not on it. Repeat several times. *Never massage the spine itself – always work at each side of it.*

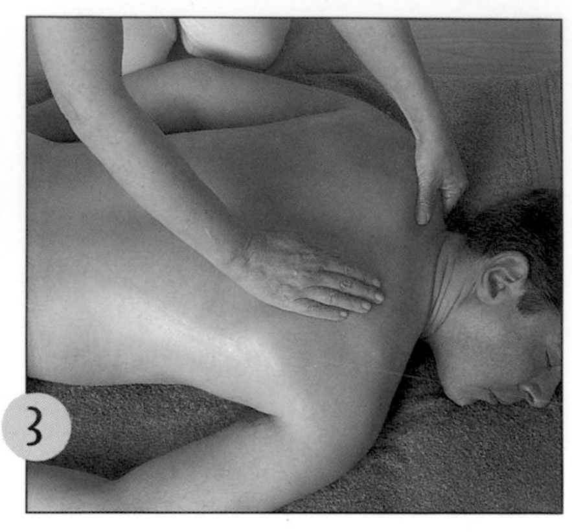

Knead the neck muscles – try to be sensitive to how your partner feels, as these muscles can often be very tense.

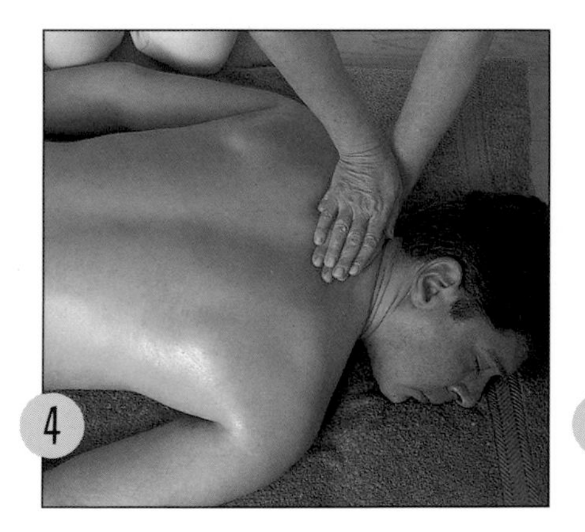

Place one hand on top of the other at the neck. This movement makes a figure-eight, and you can use the weight of your body to iron out the tension.

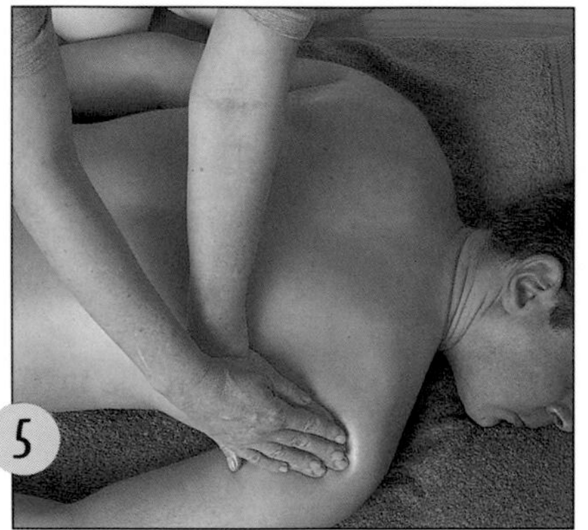

Your hands move diagonally across the back to go around the opposite shoulder blade, returning to the center and going around the first shoulder. Repeat several times.

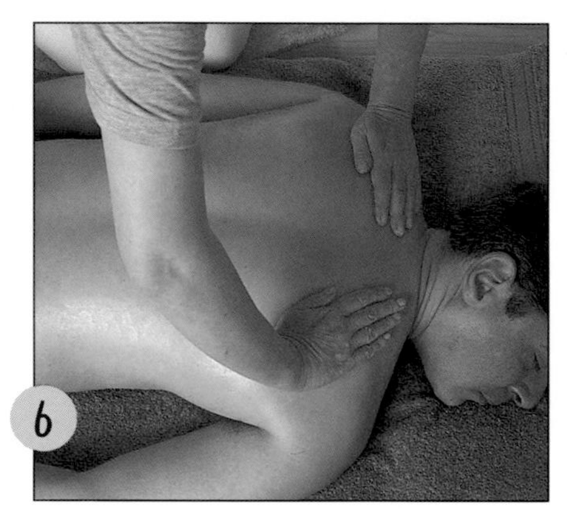

Separate your hands and do figure-eight movements over the whole surface of the back.

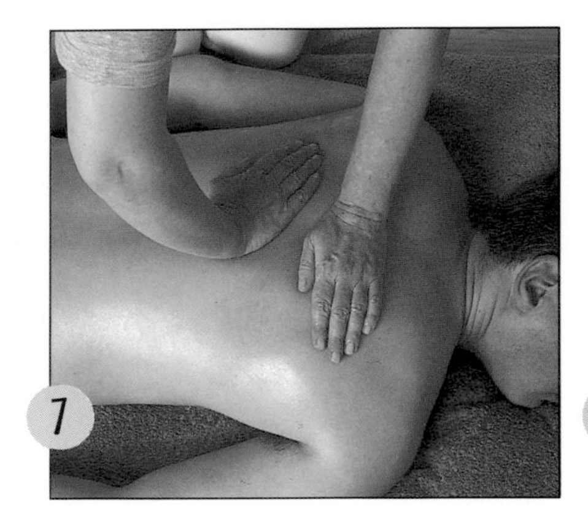

Continue this movement, traveling up and down the back, covering the whole area. Again, use your body weight in the movement.

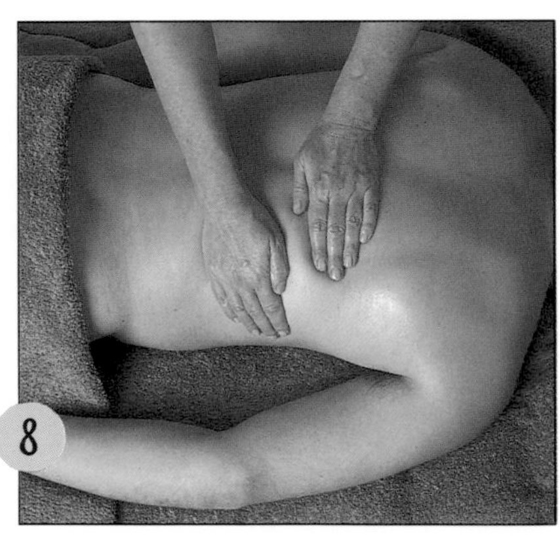

Alternate effleurage the sides of the back, starting just beneath the armpit and working down toward the waist. Change sides and repeat.

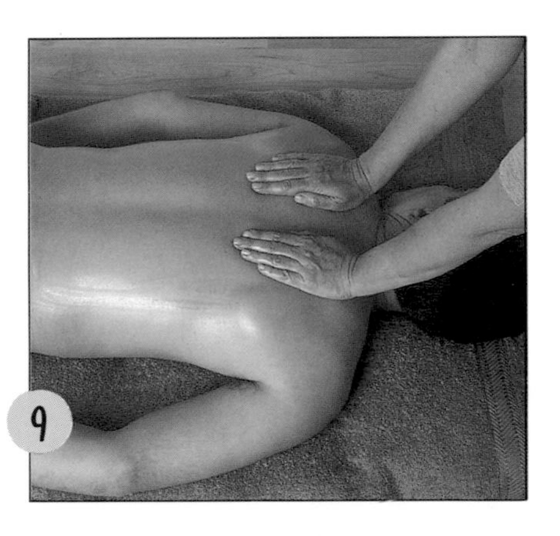

Now move around to your partner's head and effleurage down each side of the spine, again using your body weight to help release tense muscles.

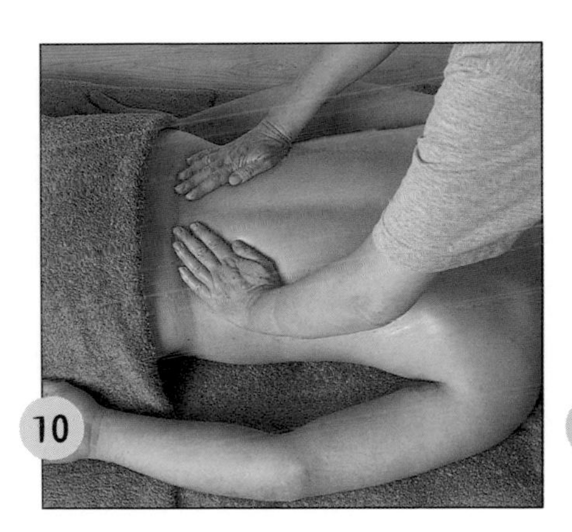

Move your hands out over the top of the buttocks and back up the sides.

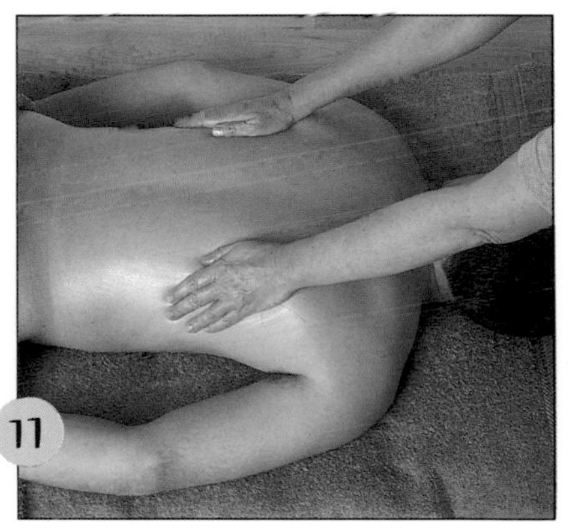

Repeat the effleurage movement several times, gradually making the pressure lighter with each repetition.

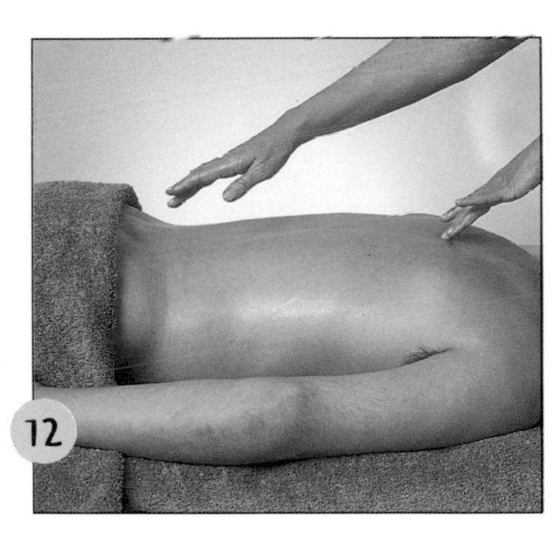

Feather-stroke from the base of the spine to the neck, again with an increasingly lighter touch. Ask your partner to turn over onto his back and rearrange the towels.

NECK AND SHOULDERS

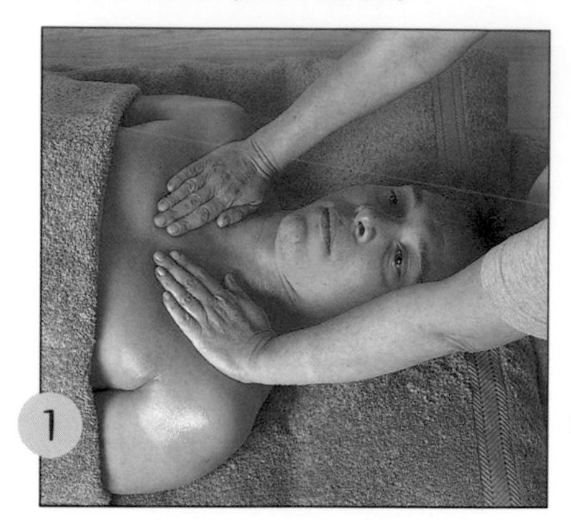

Uncover the neck and shoulders. Lay your hands flat on each side of the upper chest and simply hold them still for a few moments.

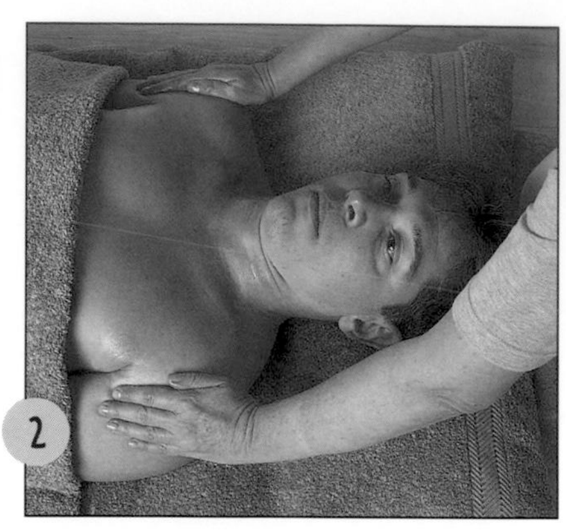

Effleurage firmly over the chest and out under the shoulders, then back up to the neck, pulling out the muscles as you do so. Repeat several times.

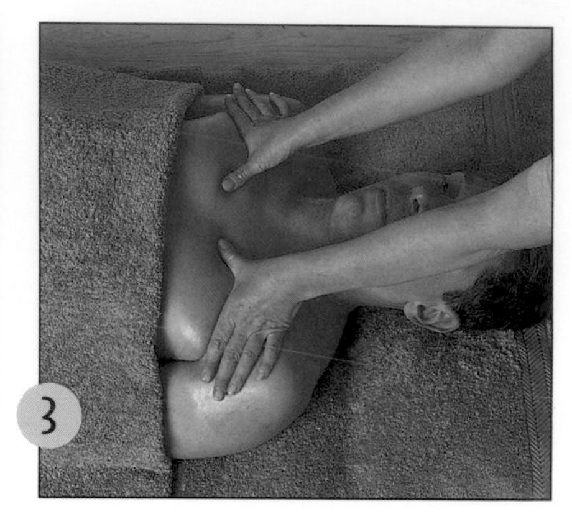

Petrissage the upper chest using the thumbs. Use a firm touch and move gradually downward.

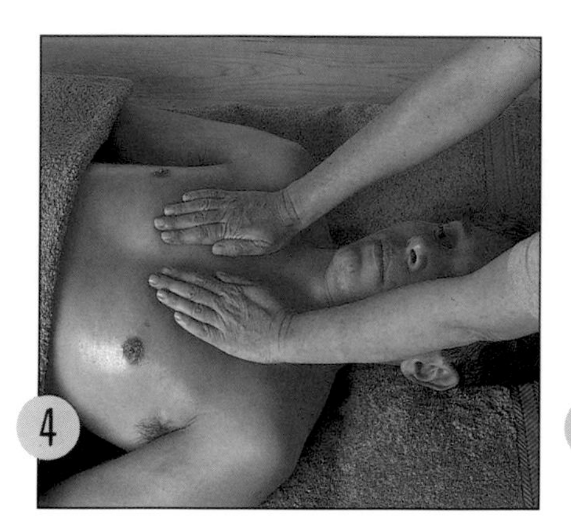

Uncover the chest and effleurage around the breasts with a firm, circular movement.

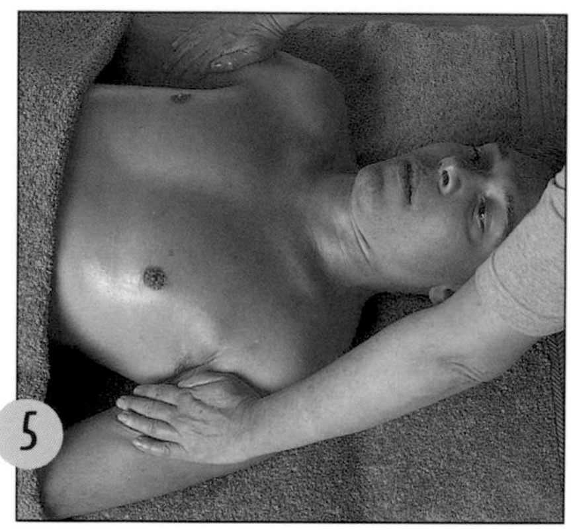

Enlarge the circle so that your hands travel out over the arms, returning up the back and coming over the shoulders.

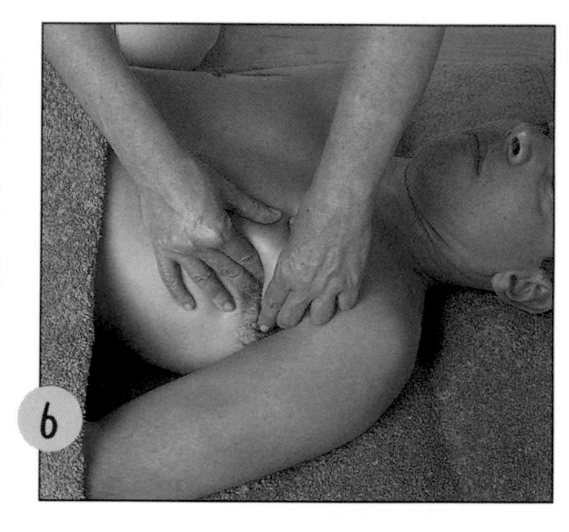

Knead the upper chest where the breast meets the armpit. Effleurage the whole area with increasing lightness of touch. Cover the chest and uncover the right arm.

ARMS, HANDS, AND WRIST

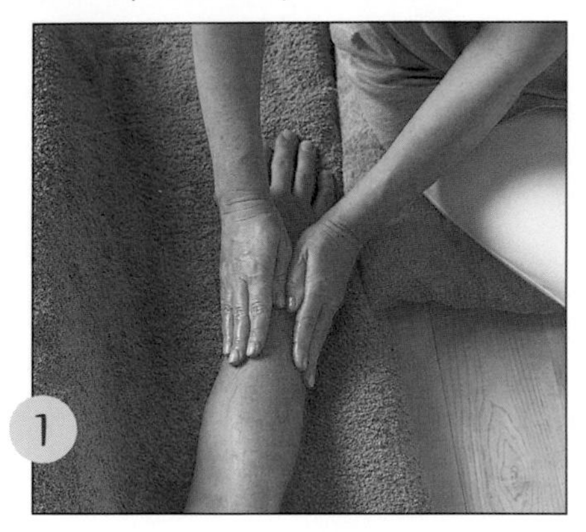

Hold the wrist in one hand and lift the arm away from the floor or bed – it should be a dead weight, with no effort made by your partner. Place your hands on each side of the wrist.

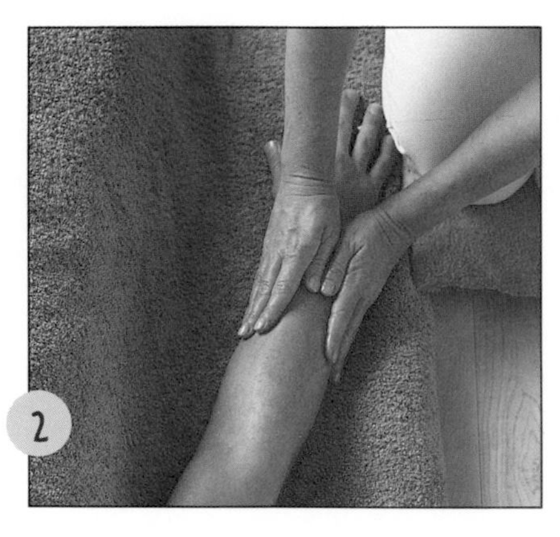

Effleurage from the wrist to the top of the arm using a firm pressure.

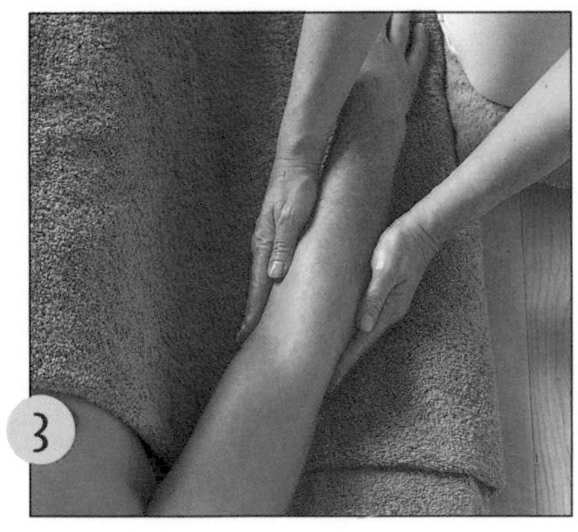

For the return movement, take your hands to the outside of the arm and sweep downward. Repeat several times.

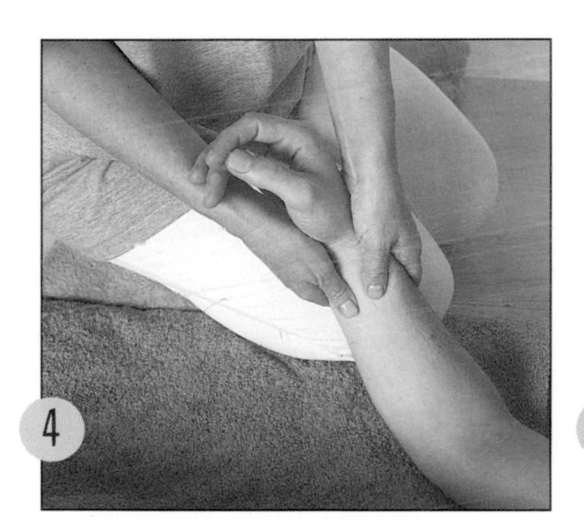

Bend the arm at the elbow with the palm uppermost. Petrissage from the wrist to the elbow, coming back down to the wrist each time in a smooth effleurage stroke. Repeat several times.

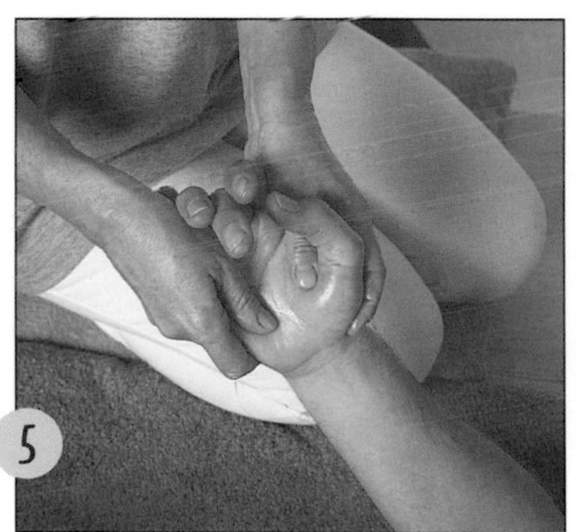

Petrissage the palm of the hand, then turn it over and petrissage very gently between the fingers.

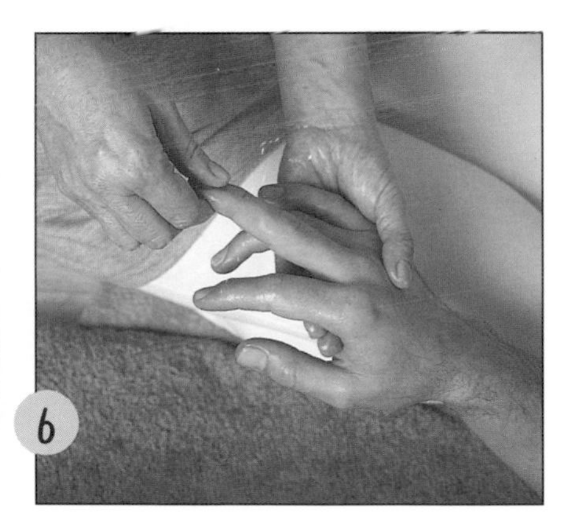

Pull each finger gently to stretch it out. Effleurage the arm as at the beginning several times. Cover it and repeat for the other arm.

Abdomen

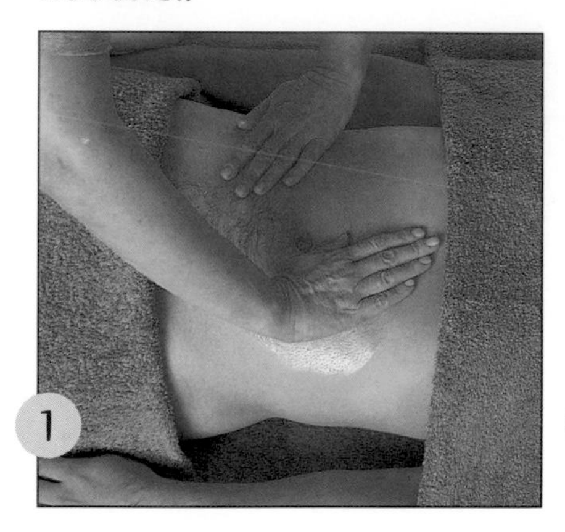

Uncover the abdomen and effleurage the whole area gently. If there is any pain here, stop immediately; do not use much pressure in any case, as this area is very sensitive.

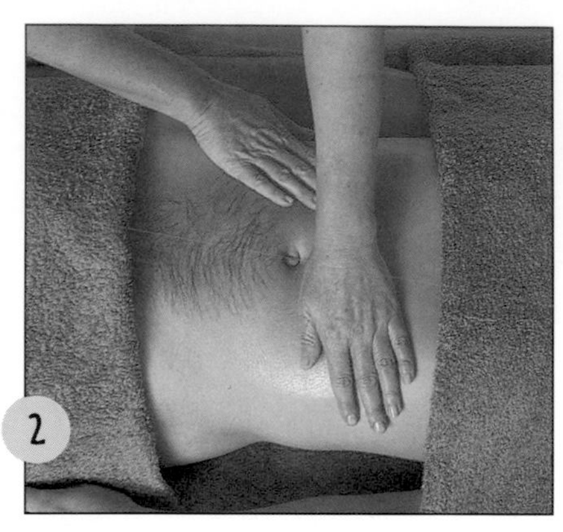

Effleurage the whole abdomen with a circular movement, one hand following the other.

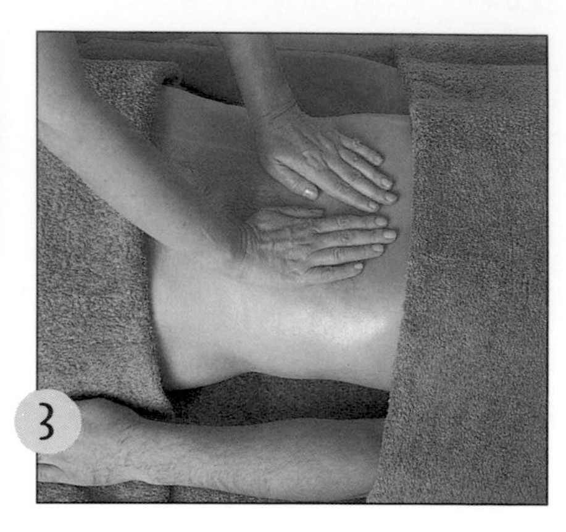

Starting with your palms together in the center of the abdomen, move them gradually apart toward the sides of the body.

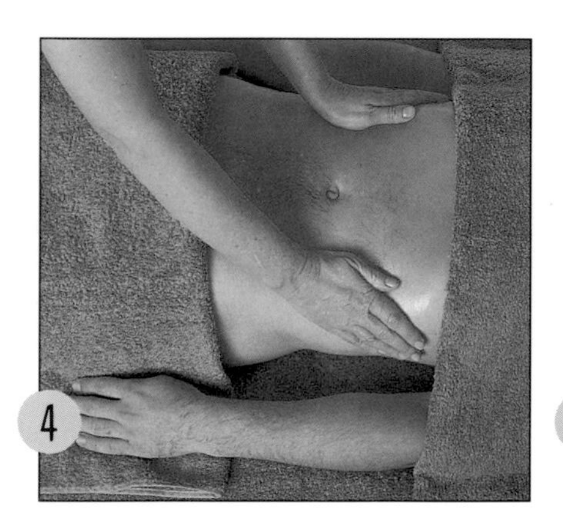

Let your hands glide out over the sides and under the back so that they just meet at the spine.

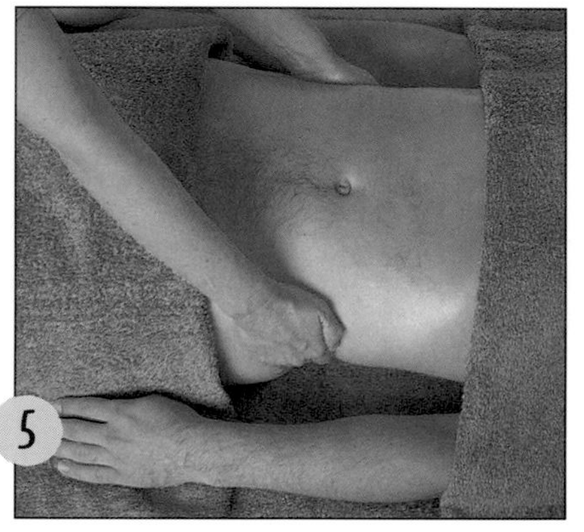

When your fingers touch beneath the back, start to draw them back, pulling out the back muscles gently as you go. Repeat several times.

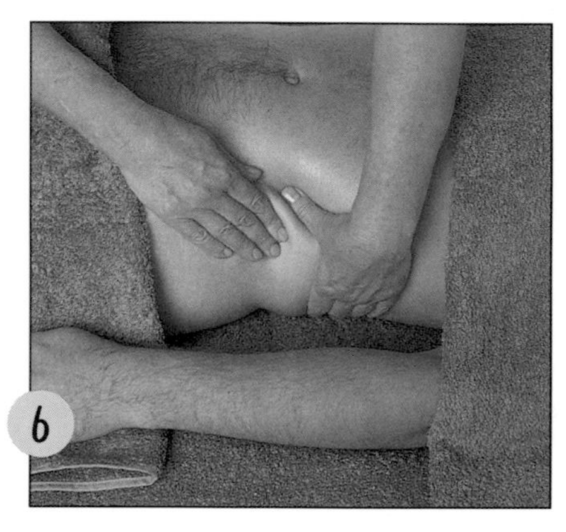

Knead one side of the abdomen, then effleurage gently. Swap sides. Cover the abdomen.

Foot, Leg, and Ankle

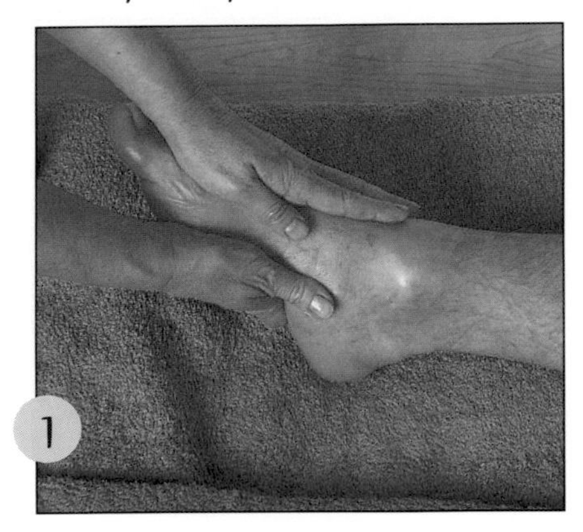

Uncover the right leg. Having warmed the oil in your palms, gently effleurage the whole of the foot.

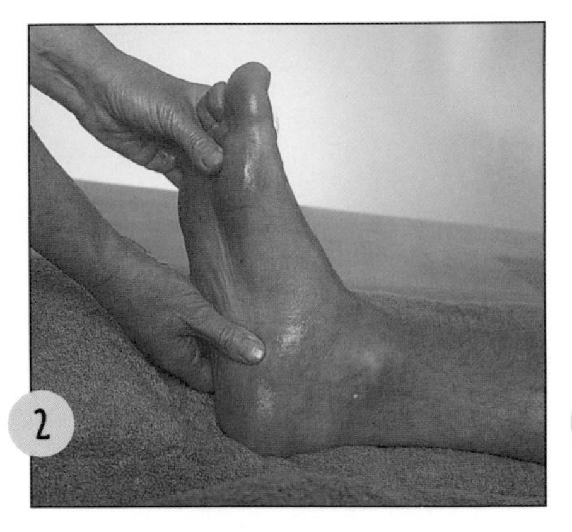

Petrissage the sole of the foot. If you use a firm pressure, this should not make your partner ticklish!

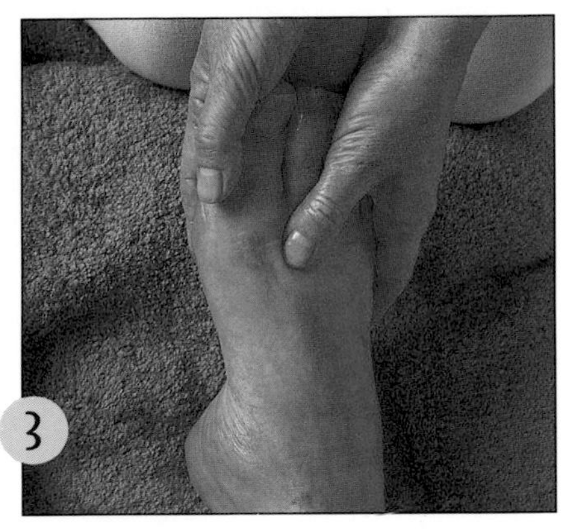

Petrissage between the toes, then pull out and gently stretch each toe.

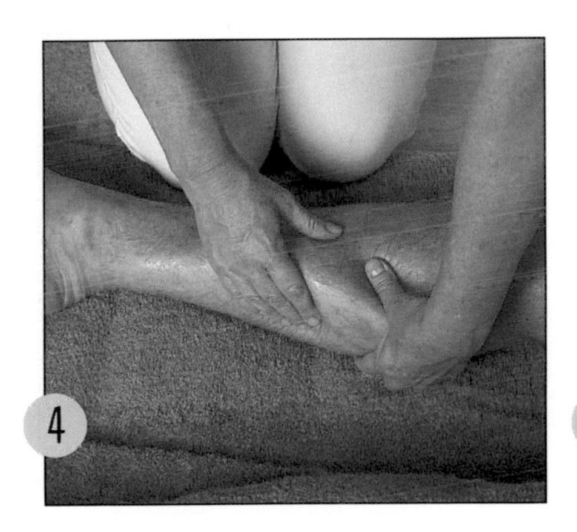

Knead the calf muscle. Effleurage from ankle to the groin, up the center, and back down the sides gently. Repeat several times. Then petrissage from the upper knee to the groin. Repeat several times.

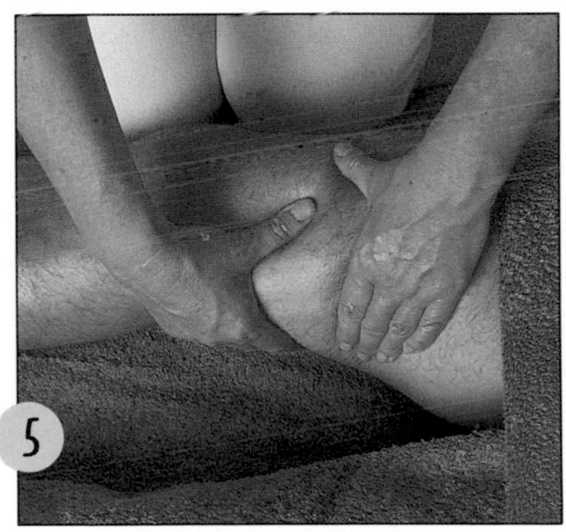

Knead the upper leg. Then alternate effleurage the whole of the upper leg. Repeat several times. Effleurage the whole leg. Cover and repeat on the left. When you have finished, cover your partner except for the feet.

Sole of Foot

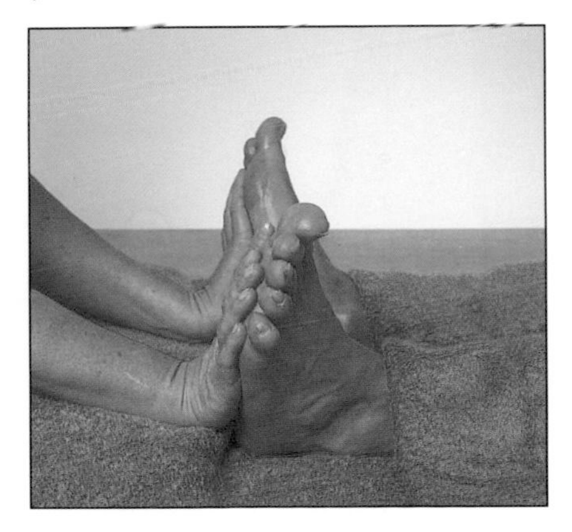

Place your palms on the soles of the feet and hold them there for at least a minute. Cover the feet and leave your partner to relax for a few minutes. Wash your hands and arms in cold water to remove negative energy.

SPECIFIC APPLICATIONS

There are a number of conditions that respond particularly well to treatment by aromatherapy. These include stress and emotional problems such as depression and insomnia; respiratory conditions, especially coughs and colds; and some digestive, muscular, and skin conditions. It can also be used as first aid for several minor emergencies, However, it is very important to recognize that aromatherapy, though very successful in some areas, has its limitations. More serious conditions – or potentially serious ones – must be treated by a doctor. The underlying rule is – if in doubt, always consult a doctor or, in an emergency, a hospital.

The uses and properties of all the aromatherapy oils are extremely complex. If you are worried by a particular condition and you decide you want to try treating it with essential oils, it is probably best in the first instance to consult a trained aromatherapist (see page 60). Nevertheless, aromatherapy can be a very useful form of home treatment and, in the following pages, various conditions are given with aromatherapy "recipes."

There is often more than one method of treating a problem – by massage or as a bath, for example. In some cases, I have given specific recipes; in others, the many oils that are beneficial for a particular condition. This gives you the basis to experiment, blending oils to produce an aroma that you like, which very often proves to be the very oil that is most beneficial. So, trust in your instincts and be creative!

A number of ailments respond well to aromatherapy oils whether used in massage, baths and compresses, or when inhaled.

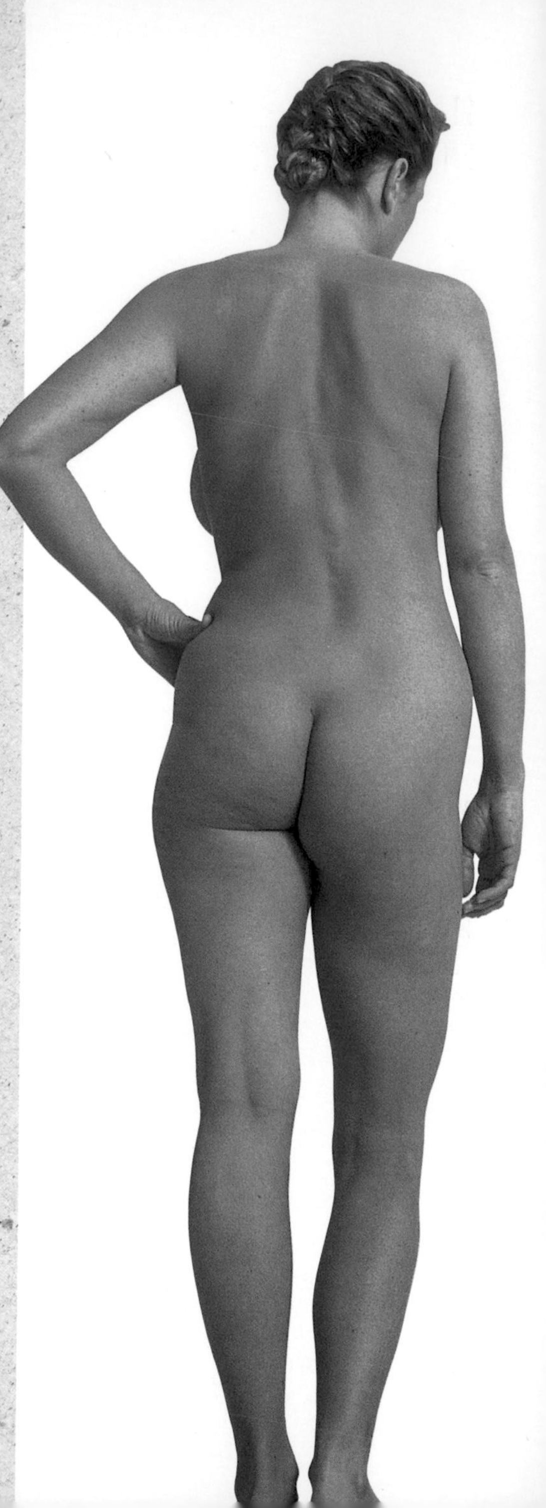

STRESS AND EMOTIONAL PROBLEMS

pages 40–42

Aromatherapy is widely recognized as an effective means of dealing with stress, particularly when combined with massage. It is also useful for other ailments which may result from an emotional cause, such as depression and insomnia.

RESPIRATORY PROBLEMS

pages 43–45

Many respiratory complaints may be relieved by inhaling essential oils, either a few drops on a pillow or tissue or as a steam inhalation. You can also massage the affected area yourself if you have a sore throat or bronchitis.

MUSCULAR AND CIRCULATORY PROBLEMS

pages 46–48

Compresses using aromatherapy oils can be particularly soothing, especially for sufferers from arthritis and rheumatism or anyone who has pain and inflammation resulting from injury.

DIGESTIVE PROBLEMS

pages 49–50

The digestive system is a delicate mechanism and, for many people, one that is particularly prone to upset. Aromatherapy oils may be useful in a wide variety of ways – from calming indigestion to relieving a hangover.

WOMEN, PREGNANCY, AND CHILDBIRTH

pages 51–53

A whole range of problems that apply specifically to women – such as PMS, menstrual cramps, and cystitis – may be effectively alleviated with essential oils. They may also prove beneficial in overcoming the side-effects experienced during pregnancy – like heartburn and morning sickness – but always check the oils to avoid in pregnancy first (see right).

SKIN AND HAIR

pages 54–56

Many skin complaints may benefit from treatment with essential oils – such as acne and eczema. Hair and scalp problems may also be improved, particularly dandruff and head lice – a common problem for schoolchildren.

CHILDREN'S PROBLEMS

page 57

Babies and children find aromatherapy oils very calming and soothing. Often the best method for them is a few drops on a pillow or in the bath water. However, if applied to the skin, always use the dosages on page 22 as young skin is very sensitive.

FIRST AID

pages 58-59

In minor emergencies, an essential oil first aid kit may prove invaluable. The oils are all antiseptic, and many have soothing and healing properties to ease burns, aches, stings, and grazes.

WARNING

There are certain contra-indications to be considered when using essential oils. For certain people or particular conditions, some oils must be avoided. These can be divided into the following groups.

Not to be used except by professional therapists

Aniseed; bay; camphor; carrot seed; hyssop; lemon grass; pennyroyal; sage; savory; tarragon; thuja; thyme; wintergreen.

Not to be used on the skin

Cinnamon (bark or leaf); cloves; rue.

Not to be used in pregnancy

Angelica; basil; cinnamon bark; clary sage; hyssop; juniper berry; lovage; myrrh; origanum; pennyroyal; rosemary; sage; savory; sweet fennel; sweet marjoram; thyme.

Children – only use the following oils

Camomile; clary sage; eucalyptus; geranium; juniper berry; lavender; peppermint; rose; rosemary; sage; sandalwood; sweet marjoram; tea tree.

Stress and Emotional Problems

One of the areas in which aromatherapy can be most advantageous is for stress and emotional problems. The oils are particularly effective for these problems when used in conjunction with a full body massage (see pages 24-37), though as a room perfume, on a pillow, in the bath water, or as a partial self-massage, they can also prove beneficial.

Fatigue and Nervous Exhaustion

Too many responsibilities – work, looking after children, running a home – and not enough time for yourself can leave you feeling it takes all your energy just to get through the day. If you do feel this way, you should try to get as much rest as possible, eat a good diet, and take regular gentle exercise – though, of course, this is easier said than done if you are starting with an impossible schedule. For an instant lift, basil oil is extremely stimulating. Used in an early morning bath or simply inhaled from a tissue during the course of the day, it can give you a boost. Rosemary, peppermint, and clary sage are also good, especially if used in the morning. Stimulating oils should be avoided at night when you need your rest. Lavender on the pillow at night helps promote a sound sleep. One of the baths or massages suggested for anxiety or insomnia is also a good way of revving down your system in the evening and preparing yourself for a good night's sleep.

Clary sage

Anxiety and Tension

Emotional tension and anxiety can hardly fail to lead to physical tension. This may result in headaches (see page 42), palpitations, various digestive disorders such as diarrhea and nausea, insomnia, and any number of other unexplained pains and problems – not to mention the possibility of long-term illnesses such as ulcers or heart disease.

The physical contact of a full body massage combined with uplifting and calming oils can help to promote much-needed relaxation. Some of the best oils for this purpose are ylang-ylang, geranium, rose, neroli, melissa, lavender, sandalwood, and patchouli. A mixture of two or three favorites can be used for a full massage by an aromatherapist or a friend, or you can use them to give yourself a mini-massage, put them in the bath water, or inhale them from a tissue by day or from your pillow at night.

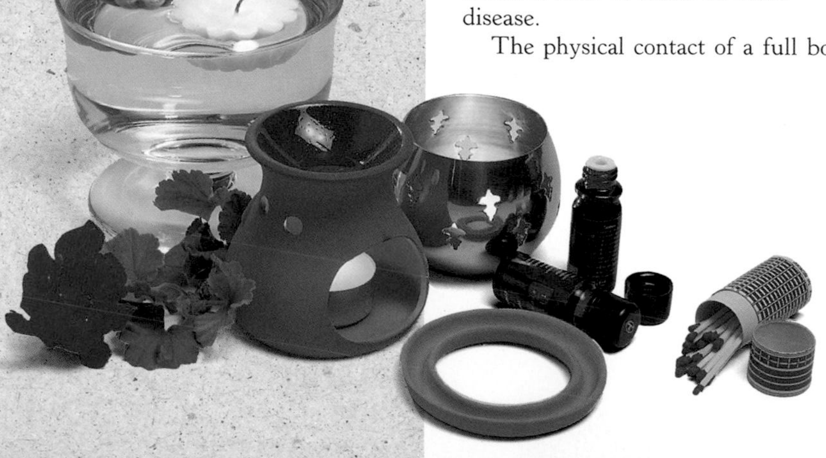

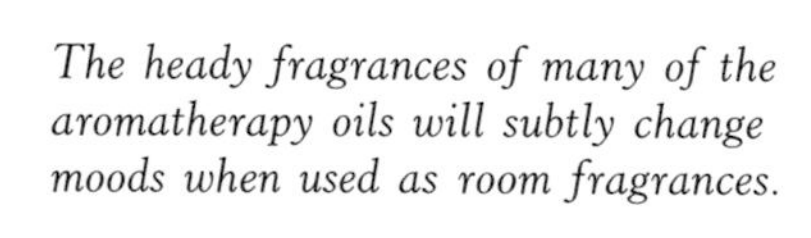

The heady fragrances of many of the aromatherapy oils will subtly change moods when used as room fragrances.

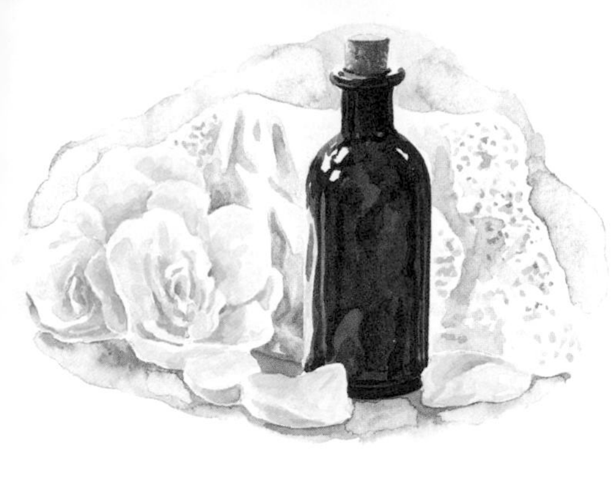

Rose or jasmine oil inhaled from a handkerchief can help to lift the spirits.

Depression

There are times when everyone feels depressed. This is often a fairly short-lived feeling, but it can develop into a chronic problem that seems impossible to overcome. Many people nowadays regard antidepressant drugs as something to be avoided at all costs and prefer to look for help elsewhere. With long-term depression, counseling may be the answer. To balance your emotional state and help you to feel able to cope, a full body massage with uplifting and relaxing oils can be beneficial. Simply the fact that it is a very pleasurable treat may help in itself. Good oils are jasmine, clary sage, ylang-ylang, bergamot, neroli, rose, orange, lemon, and lavender. Any of these oils will work well in a bath, too, and you can sprinkle a few drops of jasmine or rose on a tissue to inhale during the day.

Insomnia

Insomnia is a common result of stress, and there is nothing more frustrating than lying awake for hours, knowing you are going to feel exhausted the next, inevitably busy, day. Worrying about it, of course, only makes sleep more impossible.

Take time to wind down at the end of the day. Avoid stimulants such as coffee, and don't eat too late in the evening. Lavender, neroli, rose, and sweet marjoram are among the best oils for insomnia. They can be used for a full body massage, as a self-massage of the face, neck, and shoulders, or in the bath for a good, long soak. A few drops of lavender or neroli on your pillow is an excellent sedative and soporific.

Low Sex Drive

A low sex drive is a common result of fatigue, stress, or anxiety. It is possible to redress the sexual balance with a combination of a relaxing massage with a heady essential oil that has euphoric qualities. The best oils are rose, ylang-ylang, clary sage, patchouli, jasmine, and sandalwood, either one alone or two or three mixed together according to your own preference. You could also use one of these oils to scent a room in a vaporizer.

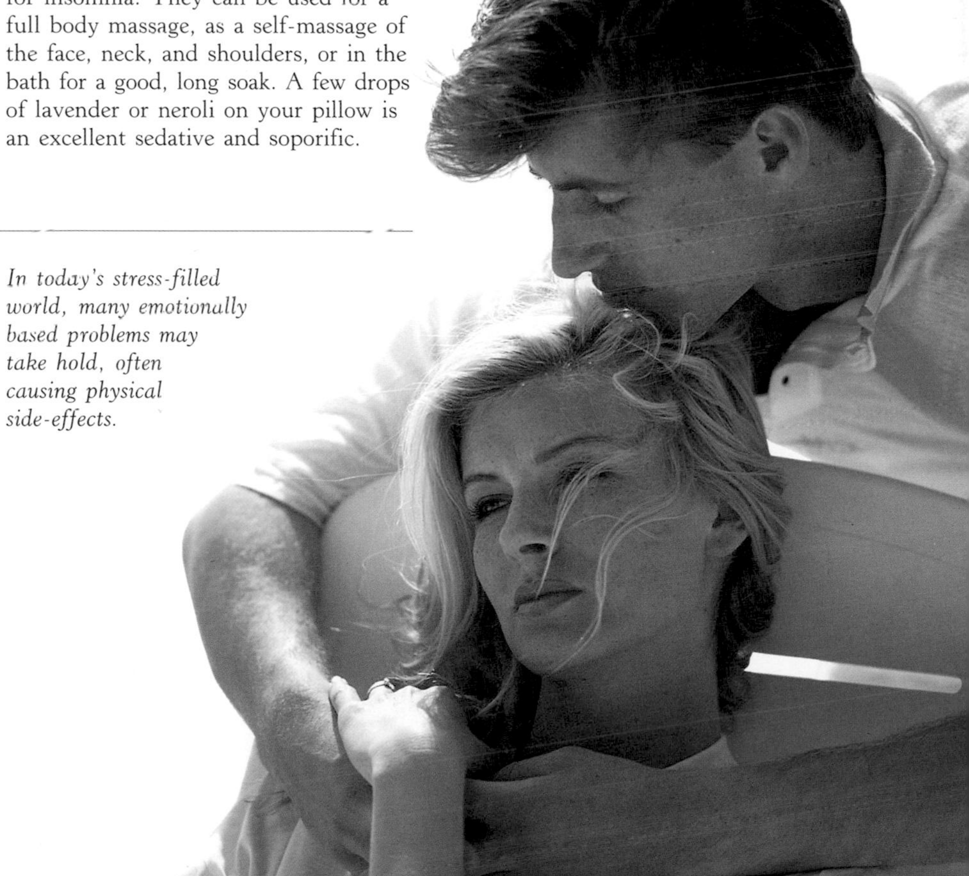

In today's stress-filled world, many emotionally based problems may take hold, often causing physical side-effects.

Headaches and Migraine

Headaches can result from stress, poor diet, hormonal disturbances, allergies, or various other factors. You should consult your doctor about severe, recurrent headaches. If it is a mild headache resulting from stress, sitting too long at your desk, or being in a noisy, smoky atmosphere, it may vanish simply by massaging a few drops of pure lavender oil into your temples and the back of your neck. Inhaling peppermint oil can sometimes bring relief, especially when massage would be painful. A neck and shoulder massage or a bath with peppermint, sweet marjoram, or melissa can also be beneficial.

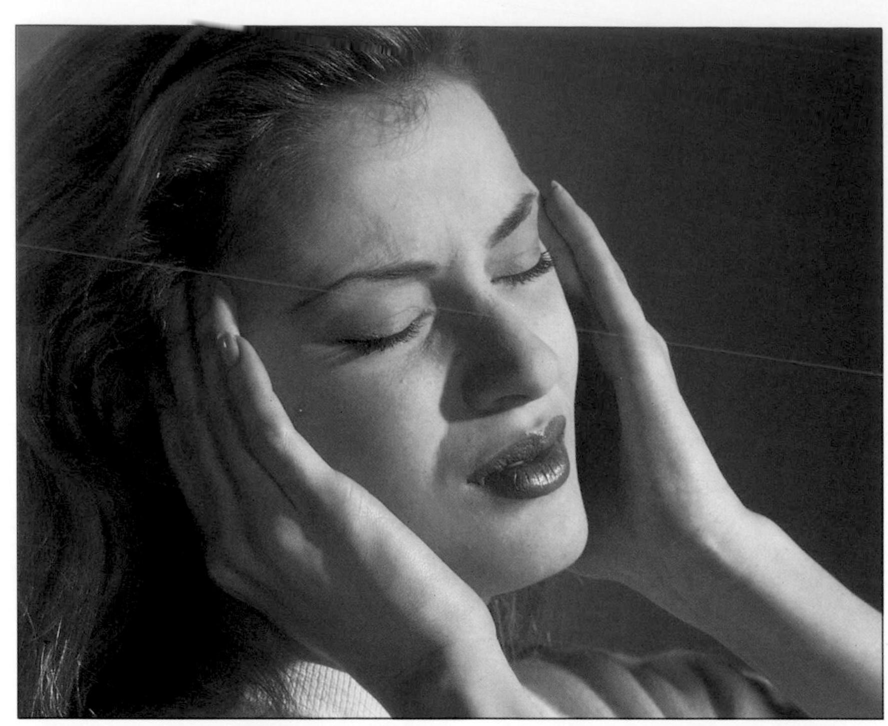

Stress headaches may be relieved simply by massaging undiluted lavender oil into the painful area.

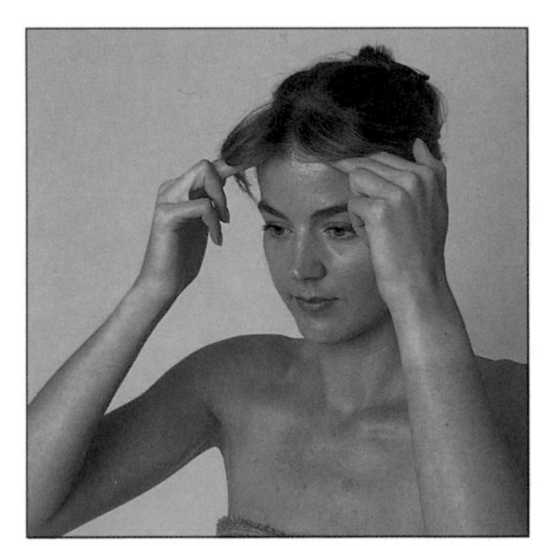

A more thorough self-massage for headache and migraine is possible. Start at the center of your forehead, at the hairline.

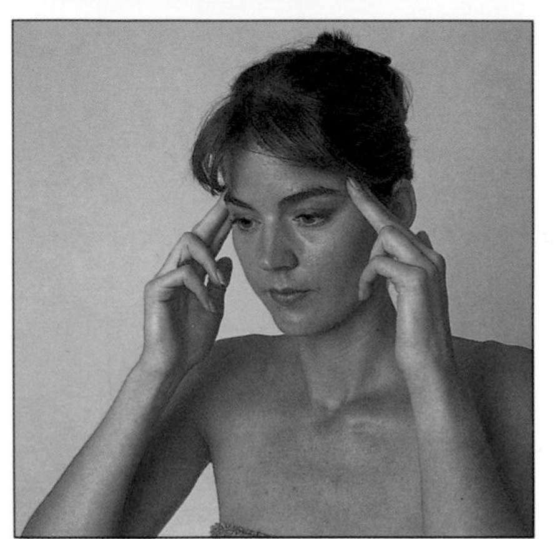

With gentle circular movements, follow the hairline around to the temples and massage this area for a few moments.

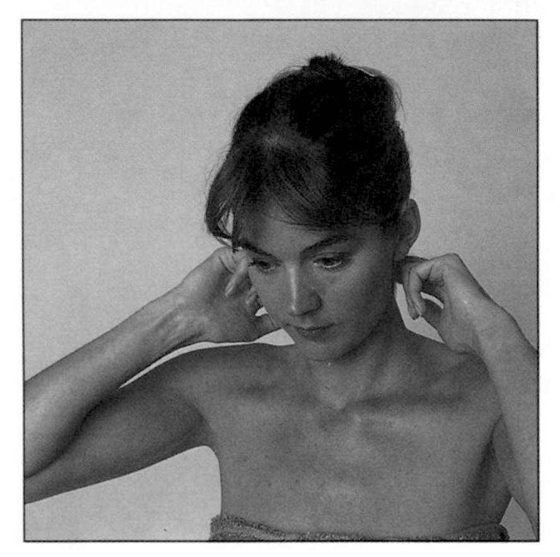

Then, continuing along the hairline, move around to the back of your neck with the same circular motion. Repeat the whole process several times.

Respiratory Problems

Because of the naturally antiseptic qualities of essential oils, their inhalation has a particularly strong and immediate effect on problems of the respiratory system. You should also make a few simple changes to your diet. If you have a cold, cough, sore throat, or flu, avoid dairy products as they produce mucus, thus aggravating the symptoms and making breathing more difficult. Avoid smoky atmospheres, and if you yourself smoke – stop!

Colds and Flu

Eucalyptus is a very important oil for problems of the respiratory tract. It is an antiseptic and decongestant, so a drop on a tissue during the day or on your pillow at night can help you to breathe and get rid of stuffiness. (It is the active ingredient in many OTC decongestants.) An inhalation of 4 drops each of tea tree and eucalyptus oils and 2 drops of peppermint in steam should be taken three or four times a day.

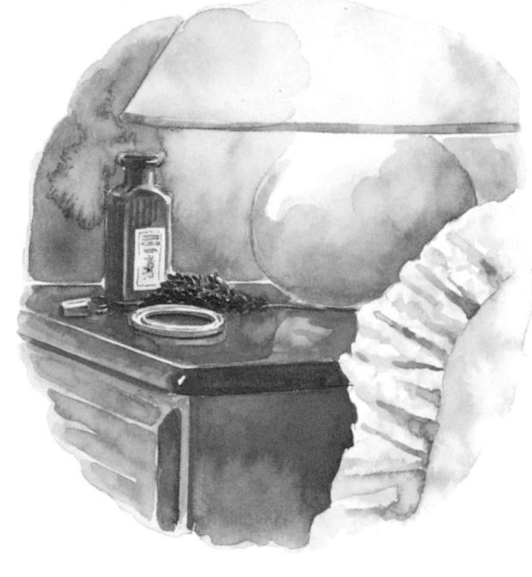

Lavender used as a room freshener has a naturally antiseptic effect, too. Gargling regularly with a drop of tea tree oil in water is a good preventative to ward off colds.

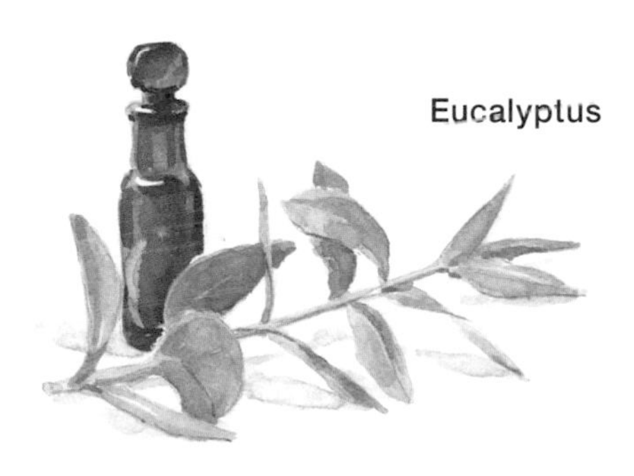

Eucalyptus

Coughs

A good mixture of oils to inhale for a cough is 4 drops each of cypress and juniper with 2 drops of ginger. For a dry cough, substitute cedarwood and camomile for the first two ingredients.

For many respiratory problems, simply inhaling an essential oil from a tissue may bring speedy relief.

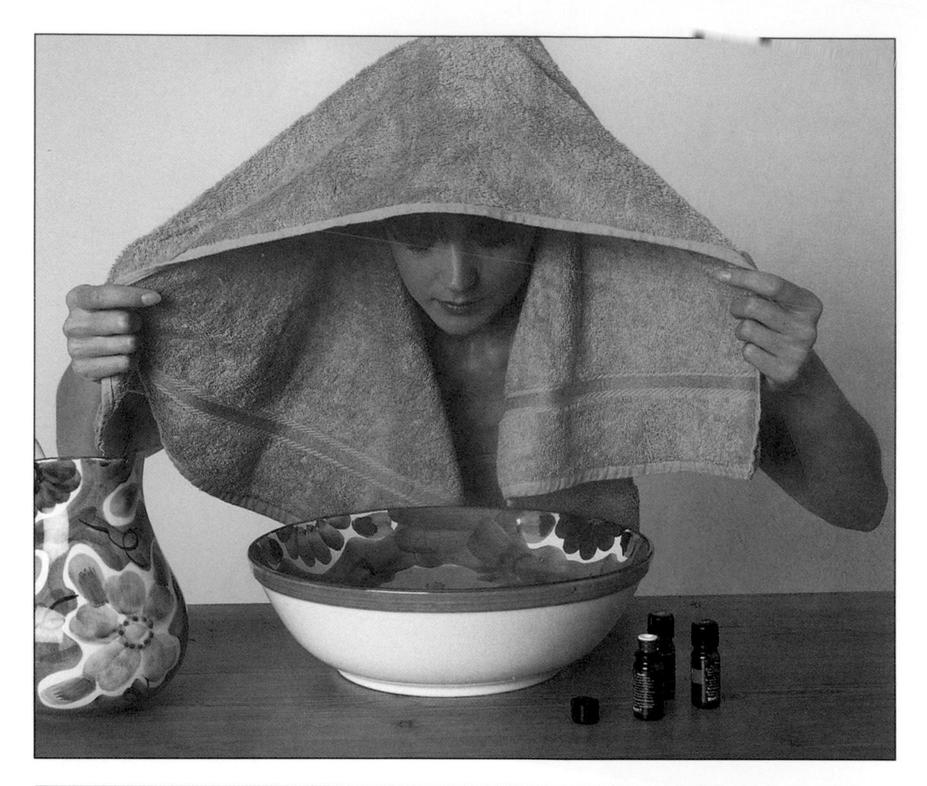

Catarrh and Sinusitis

The most common method of treatment is by steam inhalation using a mixture of 2 drops of lemon (or peppermint) oil and 4 drops each of eucalyptus and lavender oils.

You can also put the same mixture on a tissue and breathe it in regularly throughout the day. Finally, you can try a very gentle face massage, concentrating on the brow and cheekbones. Make a blend of 10 drops of lavender, 6 drops of eucalyptus, and 9 drops of peppermint in carrier oil and apply sparingly.

The symptoms of colds and flu, catarrh, and sinusitis can all be relieved by steam inhalation.

Sore Throats and Throat Infections

Gargling with 2 drops of each of tea tree and sandalwood oil in water may help to fight off a throat infection as well as bring local pain relief. It also helps laryngitis. You can apply a massage oil to the throat, face, and chest – or, better still, ask someone else to massage it for you. Mix 9 drops each of sandalwood and clary sage oils with 7 drops of ginger. You can substitute eucalyptus and peppermint for other oils in the mixture.

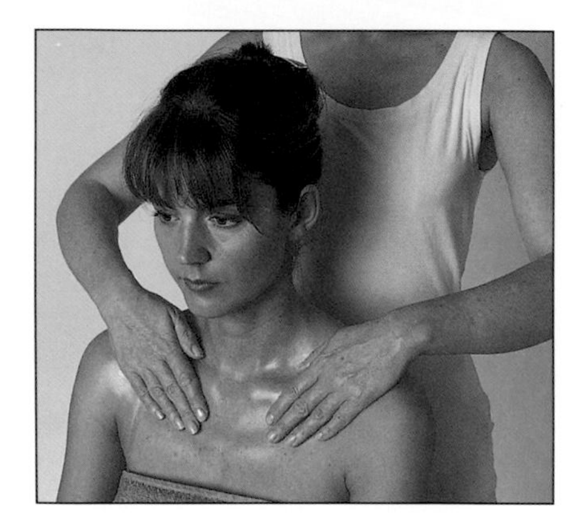

Using one of the blends mentioned left, stand behind your partner and put your hands flat on the top of her chest. Leave them there for a minute, then make long sweeping strokes across and up the chest.

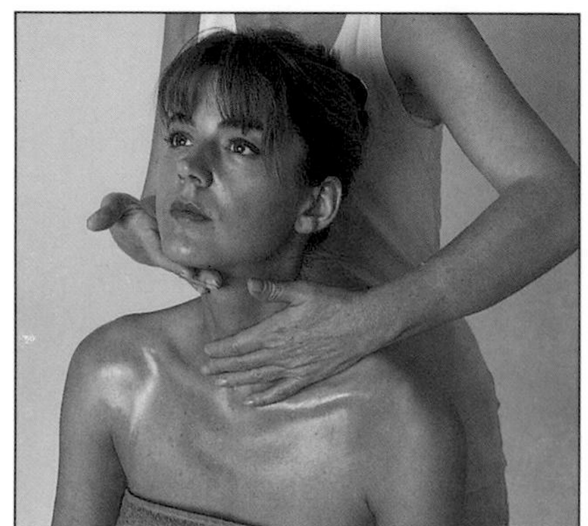

Continue the strokes up the throat toward the chin. When you have finished, wrap your partner up in towels to rest for half an hour while the oil is absorbed into her skin.

Tonsillitis

Consult a doctor about an attack of tonsillitis whether in adults or children. A steam inhalation with bergamot may bring some relief for adults.

Bergamot

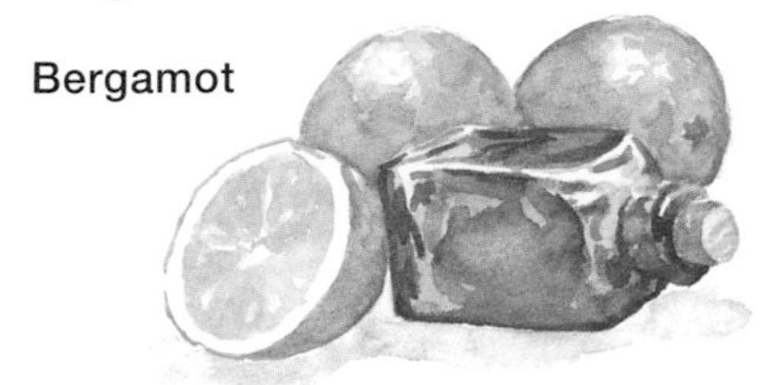

Earache

Sinusitis can cause earache as a side-effect. A compress of either lavender or camomile laid over the painful area should bring relief.

Use natural cotton fabric to make a compress. Soak it in hot water to which lavender or camomile oil has been added and apply it to the skin for at least one hour.

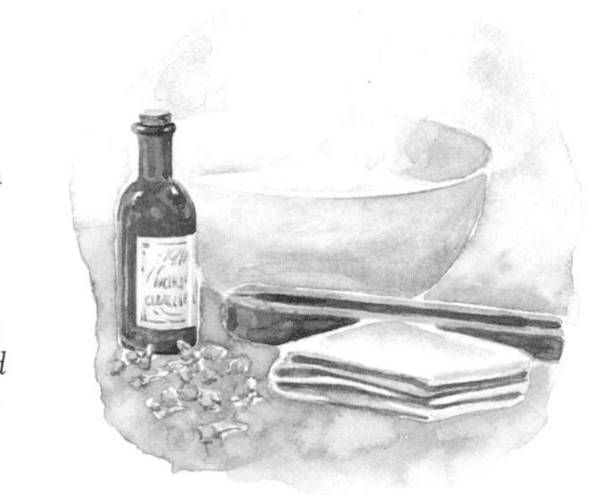

Asthma

Again, consult your doctor about this problem. However, you can try inhaling from a tissue – though not over steam – a few drops of lavender, sage, eucalyptus, or frankincense oil. You can experiment to find a blend that suits you and use the same mixture in carrier oil for massage, which feels especially good on the chest and back.

Bronchitis

Consult your doctor about bronchitis. For temporary relief, try a steam inhalation of 4 drops each of cedarwood and eucalyptus oils with 2 drops of sandalwood. You can also massage the chest and throat with the same oils diluted in carrier oil in the proportion 10:10:5.

Cedarwood, eucalyptus, or sandalwood oils are suitable for temporary relief from bronchitis.

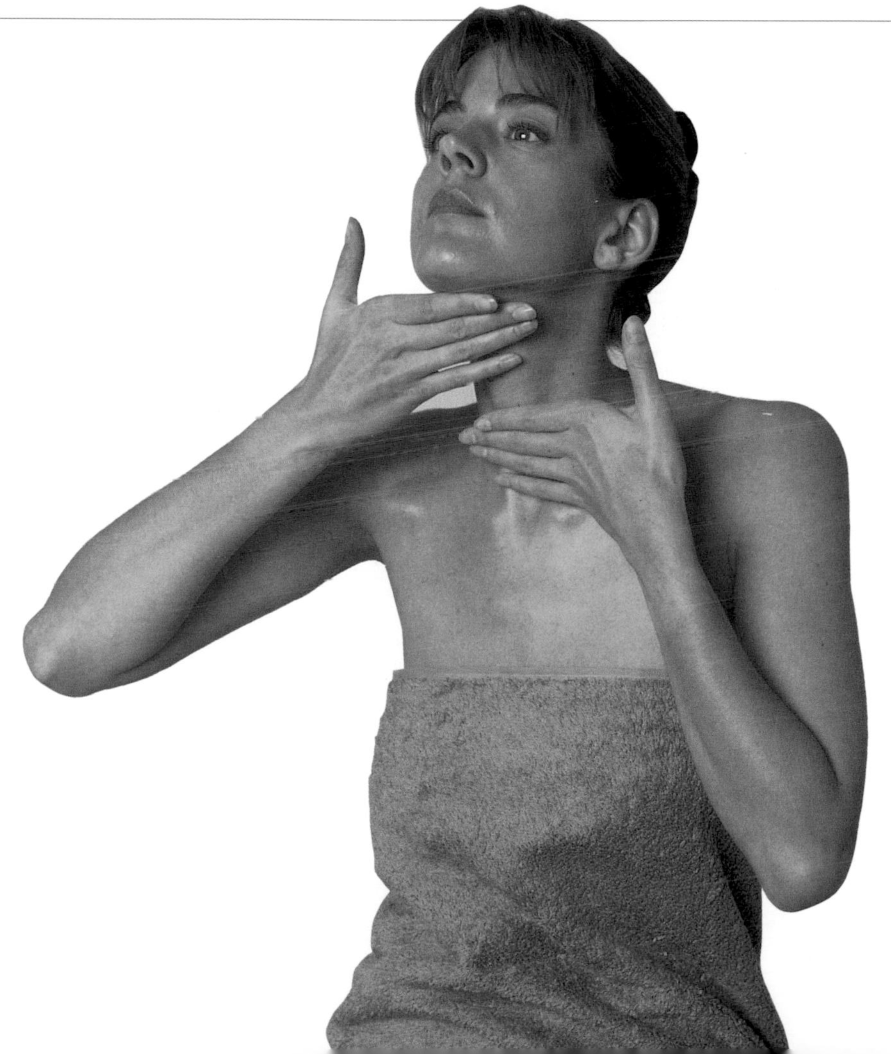

A chest and throat massage with cedarwood, eucalyptus, and sandalwood oils will relieve the uncomfortable symptoms of bronchitis.

MUSCULAR AND CIRCULATORY PROBLEMS

Backache is one of the commonest problems in western society. It can be the result of injury, poor posture, weak supporting muscles, even stress. Sports injuries are another common complaint and both respond well to essential oils, especially when they are combined with massage.

Rheumatism and arthritis are problems we usually associate with the elderly, but in fact, they can affect people of any age, including children. If there is pain or inflammation, avoid massage, however, and use compresses or baths instead.

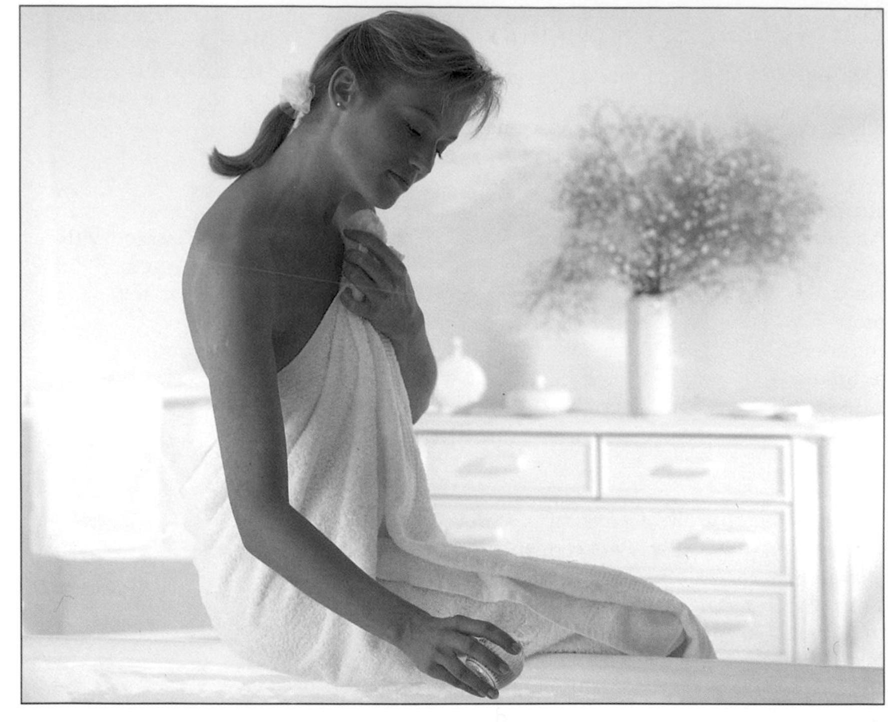

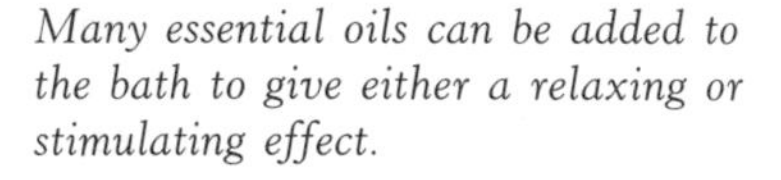

Many essential oils can be added to the bath to give either a relaxing or stimulating effect.

RHEUMATISM AND ARTHRITIS

Rheumatism is the lay term for pain and stiffness in the muscles and joints; arthritis for pain and swelling in the joints. Osteoarthritis, a degenerative disease of the joints, wears away the protective cartilage, often of the fingers, knees, hips, and spine. There can be severe pain and swelling leading to immobility. Aromatherapy is helpful as a pain relief and muscle relaxant. If joints are swollen and painful, baths and compresses should be used instead of massage. Try a blend of two or three of these oils as a compress or in a bath – camomile, pine, eucalyptus, lavender, juniper, ginger, rosemary, lemon, and sweet marjoram. If massage would not be painful – and inflamed joints must *always* be avoided – a blend of 10 drops each of rosemary and frankincense with 5 drops of eucalyptus can be made with half the usual amount of carrier oil (1oz.).

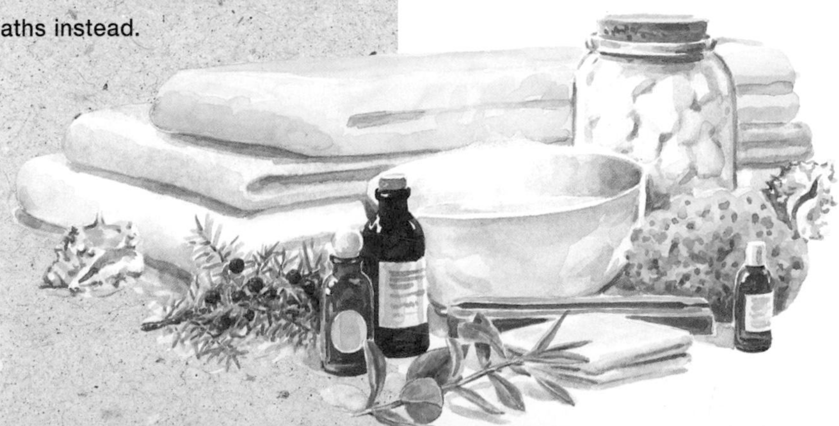

MUSCULAR ACHES AND PAINS (INCLUDING BACKACHE)

These may be general aches and pains caused by physical exertion (perhaps in sport), extreme tiredness, or a side-effect of another ailment such as flu. Alternatively, you may have a long-term back problem resulting from an old injury or because of postural problems. If the latter is the cause, consider yoga or the Alexander technique as a long-term option.

Massage may be beneficial in all of these cases, but it should be very gentle, particularly if there is any inflammation or a muscle is tensed. Remember that, in back massage, the spine itself is not touched – only massage at its sides.

You can massage the afflicted area or have a whole body massage with a mixture of 12 drops of ginger, 5 drops of juniper, and 8 drops of rosemary or lavender (rosemary is more invigorating, lavender more soothing). A bath or a compress using camomile, lavender, juniper, eucalyptus, or rosemary may also be beneficial.

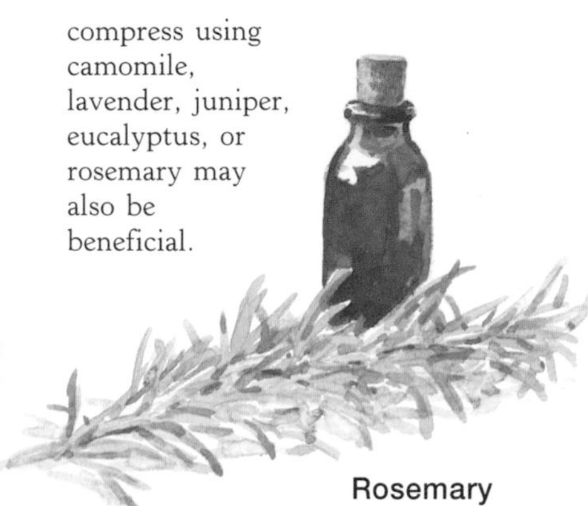
Rosemary

CRAMP

This may be a result of physical exertion, in which case the treatment is the same as for muscular aches and pains. Some people, however, suffer from long-term recurrent cramps. I treated one elderly man who would wake several times every night with cramps in his feet and legs. He found that a twice-weekly foot massage gave him an uninterrupted sleep and no pain. I used a mixture of 10 drops each of lavender and rosemary and 5 drops of sweet marjoram.

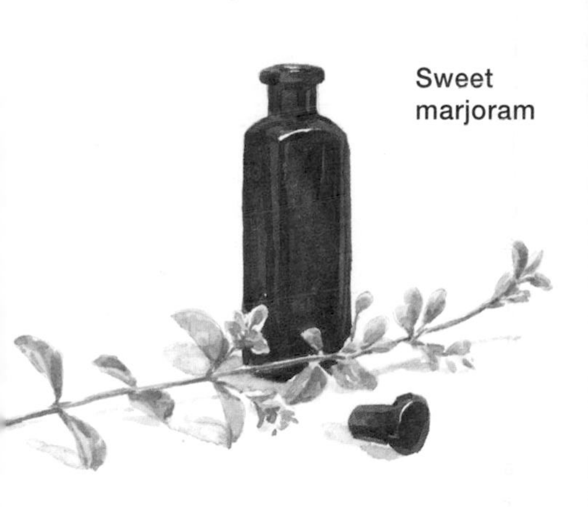
Sweet marjoram

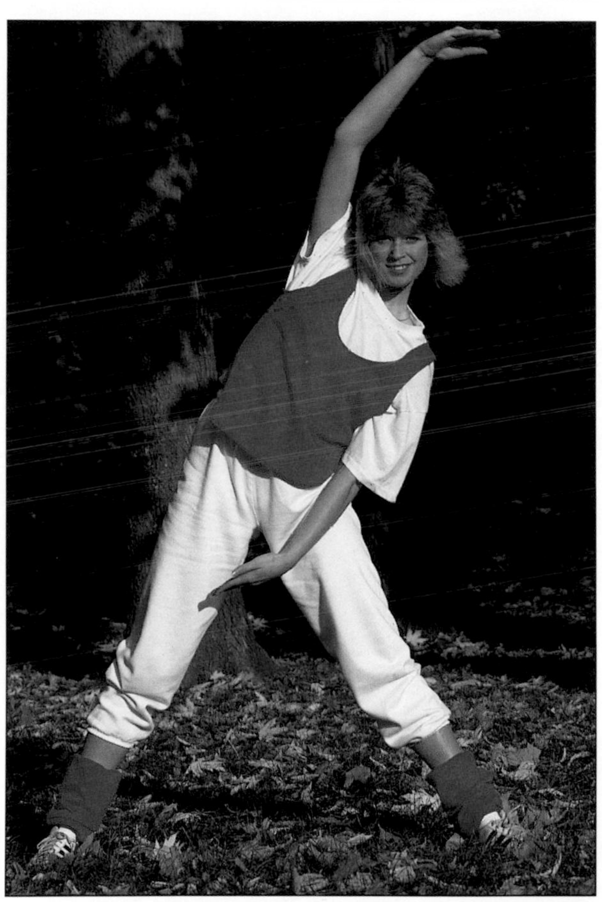
While regular exercise has an overall beneficial effect, there is always the risk of injury or just general aches and pains resulting from unaccustomed exertion. Baths and massage can both be of help in different circumstances.

Poor Circulation and Low Blood Pressure

Circulation can be improved by taking gentle exercise and also by deep breathing exercises. Massage and baths with essential oils may also be beneficial, and stimulating essences such as juniper, cypress, black pepper, rosemary, orange, and lemon are recommended. Mix two or three together according to your personal preference.

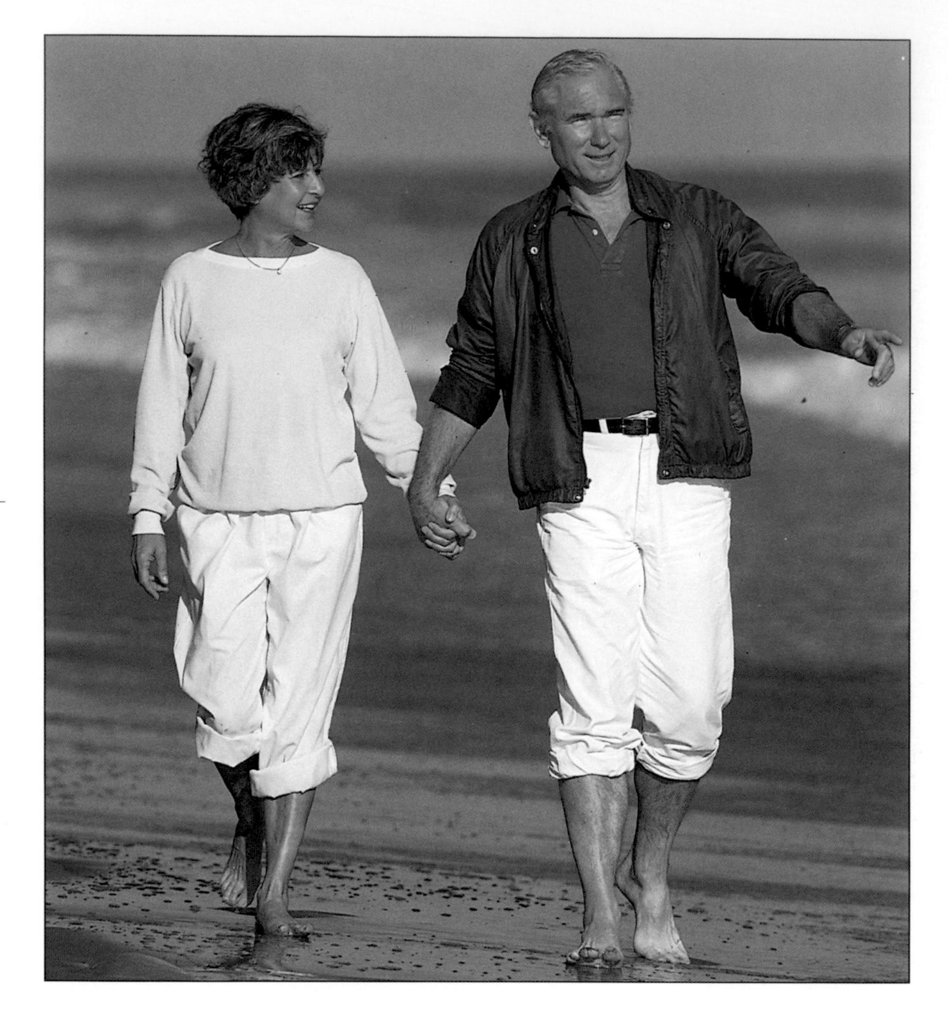

Exercise, especially when taken in the fresh air, improves circulation, as well as having an overall stimulating effect.

Varicose Veins and Hemorrhoids

Varicose veins often occur during pregnancy, but they do affect both men and women, with the veins in the legs becoming swollen and knotted. Walking as often as possible is recommended. Hemorrhoids are varicose veins that occur inside or outside the anus. They can be painful and bleed during a bowel movement. Constipation (page 50) is a common cause.

Warm (not hot) baths with cypress oil are recommended for both problems. For varicose veins, a blend of cypress, lemon, and lime can be used as a massage oil. Sandalwood may also be used.

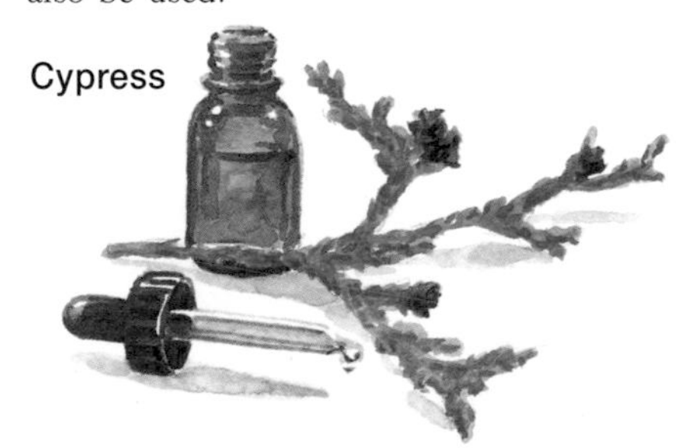

Cypress

High Blood Pressure

High blood pressure can also be improved by making some adjustments to your day-to-day habits. Cutting out smoking and heavy drinking, and changing to a healthier diet may all help, as may relaxation techniques if you are suffering from stress. You should also consult your doctor. Aromatherapy is particularly useful in this context as a whole body massage to facilitate deep relaxation, using oils such as ylang-ylang, lavender, lemon, and sweet marjoram – two or three mixed according to personal preference.

DIGESTIVE PROBLEMS

The digestive system is a delicate mechanism for many people and the place in which symptoms of stress manifest themselves – especially nausea and diarrhea. Constipation is an extremely widespread problem in western societies – principally due to diet.

Large quantities of fresh (preferably raw) fruit and vegetables, together with drinking plenty of water, are basic essentials for a good diet and a healthy digestive system.

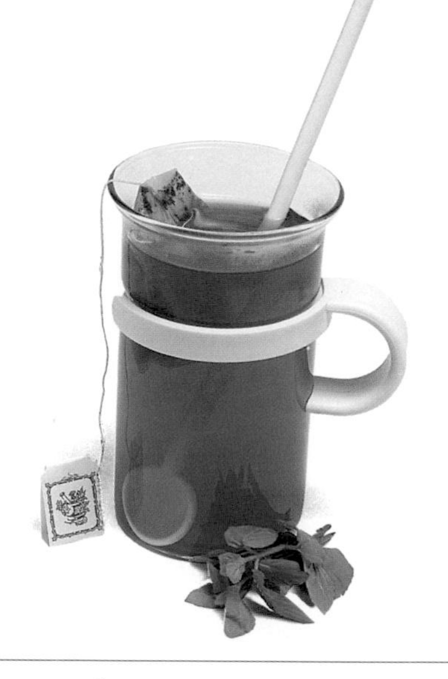

INDIGESTION, NAUSEA, AND FLATULENCE

One of the best oils for digestive problems is peppermint. For indigestion, nausea, or flatulence, drink a glass of honey water with 4 drops added. Alternatively, for indigestion, you could gently massage a blend of 10 drops each of peppermint and ginger and 5 drops of lemon in 50ml of carrier oil into the abdomen. Peppermint and camomile herbal teas are also useful.

Peppermint and camomile tea may help relieve symptoms of digestive problems.

CANKER SORES

Canker sores can appear on the gums, cheeks, or along the edges of the tongue because of stomach upsets or poor diet. However, they often occur as a result of stress, too. You can apply undiluted oils to them or use a mouthwash. If applying directly, alternate every 3 or 4 hours with 1 drop of myrrh or tea tree oil on a cotton swab.

As a mouthwash, you can mix together 1 drop each of tea tree, geranium, lavender, and lemon oils in a glass of water and use every 2 hours.

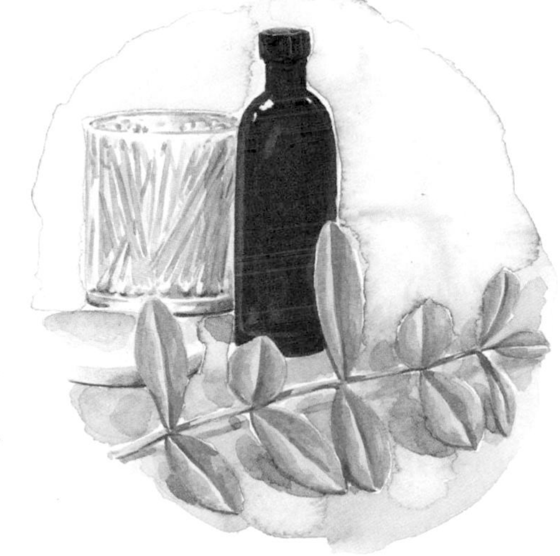

Apply pure tea tree or myrrh oil directly onto the canker sore with a cotton swab for relief from symptoms.

HANGOVER

If you wake up with a hangover, the most important aid to recovery is water – drink plenty of it and add 1 drop of rose or peppermint oil to each glass, and a teaspoon of honey. A compress using geranium oil may help a thumping head, and for a restorative bath, add 2 drops each of lavender and juniper oils and 1 drop of rosemary.

Geranium

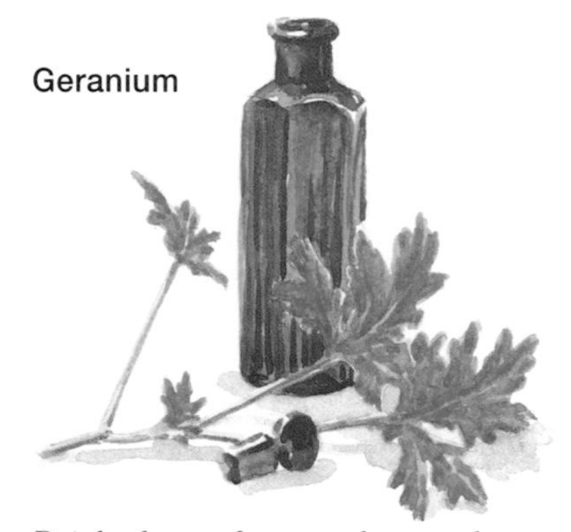

Drink plenty of water when you have a hangover, adding just one drop of rose or peppermint oil and a teaspoon of honey.

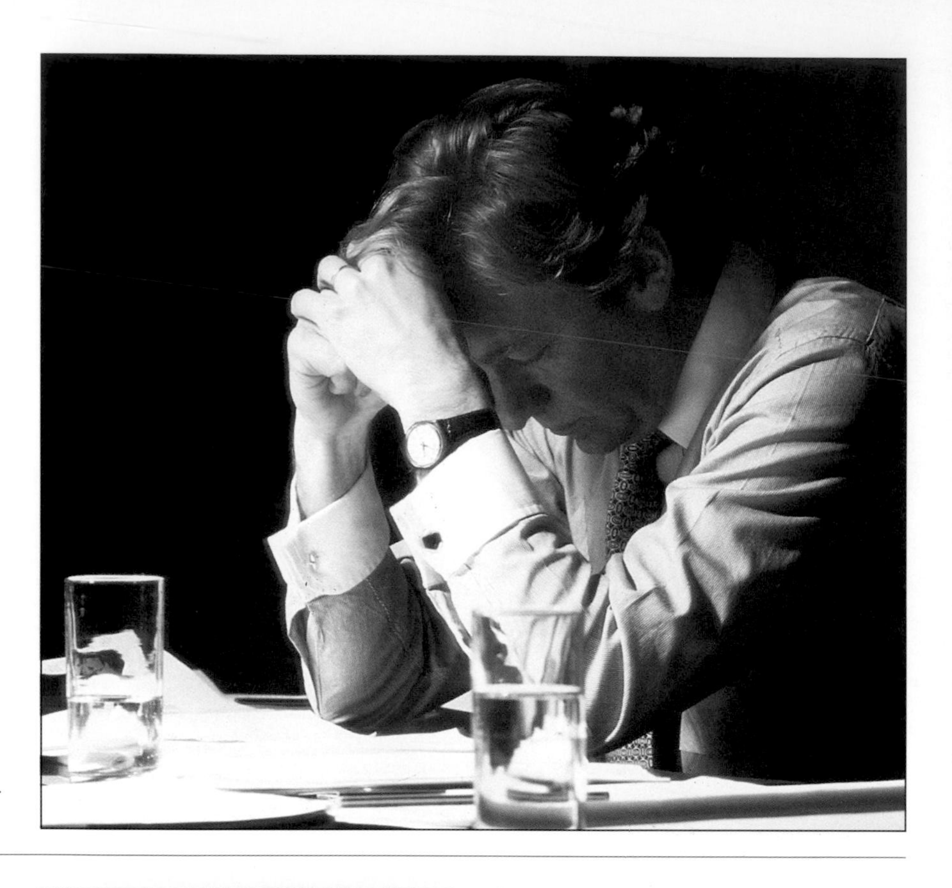

CONSTIPATION

Constipation must be addressed taking overall diet, fiber intake, and exercise into consideration, and you may need to consult your doctor if this is a long-term problem. If you suffer occasionally from mild constipation, this is a useful blend to massage into the lower back, buttocks, and abdomen: 10 drops each of marjoram and rosemary, 5 drops of black pepper.

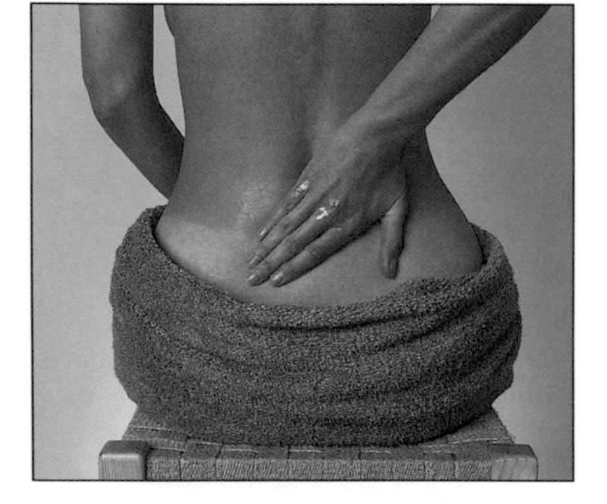

Massaging the lower back with a marjoram, rosemary, and black pepper blend can be useful for mild constipation.

DIARRHEA

Diarrhea can result from a number of causes – anything from stress to food poisoning. It can even be a side-effect of jetlag. See your doctor if the problem lasts for more than a day or so. You may find a bath with 2 drops of geranium, juniper berry, and peppermint oils added will ease the problem. Alternatively, massage the abdomen very gently in a clockwise direction with a blend of 5 drops each of peppermint, tea tree, sandalwood, and geranium oils in the usual 2 oz. (50ml) of carrier oil. This can also be rubbed gently into the lower back.

WOMEN, PREGNANCY, AND CHILDBIRTH

The delicacy and complexity of the female reproductive system leaves it open to many problems, and few women manage to get through life without suffering from period cramps, PMS, or unpleasant menopausal symptoms. Much of this may be relieved by the use of aromatherapy oils. Many of the side-effects of pregnancy, too, may be alleviated – such problems as stretch marks, nausea in the morning, backache (see page 47), and heartburn. However, great care must be taken with essential oils during pregnancy – check the list on page 39 before use.

MENSTRUAL CRAMPS

Many women suffer from painful period cramps and often experience up to 48 hours of misery. The best mixture I have found is an oil made up of 5 drops each of camomile and geranium and 15 drops of clary sage. Sweet marjoram can also be used, but the most important oil in the mixture is the clary sage. Massage the oil into the abdomen on the flat of your hand in a circular motion (going clockwise as you look down). You may also find it effective to massage some of the oil into the small of the back.

You can take clary sage oil internally as well, using 3 drops in a glass of water.

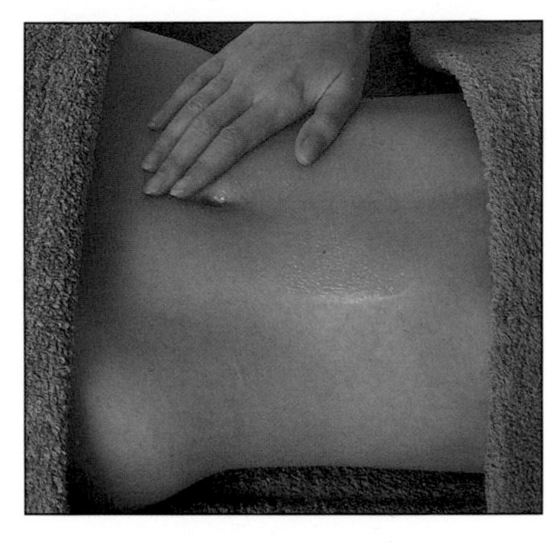

A gentle massage – in a clockwise direction – of the abdomen with clary sage, camomile, and geranium can be effective in relieving menstrual cramps.

PMS

If you get irritable or depressed just before the onset of your period, the easiest way to calm and uplift the spirits is in a bath to which ylang-ylang and clary sage have been added. If you have an aromatherapist or a friend who can give you a whole body massage, this is better still. Use the same oils in roughly equal proportions.

CYSTITIS

Caused by an inflammation of the lining of the bladder, cystitis can be a particularly painful and distressing problem. Not only does it make you want to rush to the bathroom every few minutes, there is a burning sensation when you urinate.

Internally, you can take one drop of camomile oil in a glass of honey water. You can also take two baths a day (at least) staying in for between 10 and 15 minutes. Add 2 drops of lavender, juniper berry, eucalyptus, and sandalwood oils. It is very important to drink as much uncarbonated spring water as possible, too.

It is very important to drink as much uncarbonated spring water as possible with cystitis. You can also take internally a drop of camomile oil in honey water.

Yeast

The white and sometimes smelly discharge of yeast is a result of the intestinal fungus, *candida albicans*, multiplying out of control. It is a very common problem, and many women find it a particularly embarrassing one. Regular baths with 2 drops each of tea tree, myrrh, and bergamot oils may bring some relief.

Cellulite

Massage roughly equal proportions of juniper, rosemary, and lavender oils into affected areas on the thighs, hips, and buttocks. You should use firm strokes, moving up from the knee, but no pummeling.

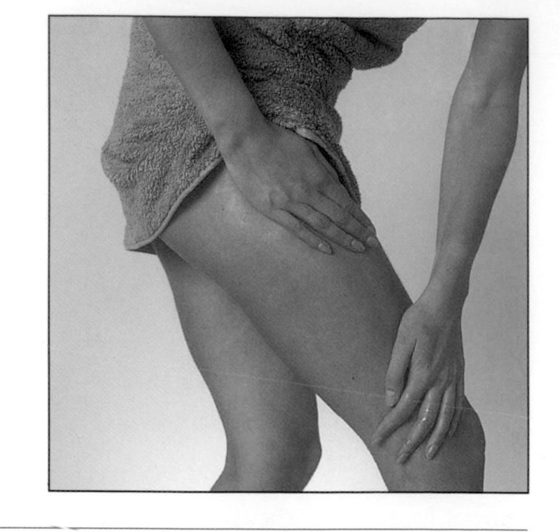

Massage areas of cellulite on a regular daily basis with a blend of juniper, rosemary, and lavender oils.

Stretch Marks

Although they are usually associated with pregnancy, stretch marks can also be caused by extreme overweight. They will never disappear, but massaging with a blend of 20 drops of lavender and 5 of neroli (preferably in a rich carrier oil such as wheatgerm or almond) will improve them. This is a good mixture to use from the fourth month of pregnancy as a preventative, too. Apply morning and night to the abdomen, thighs, and breasts.

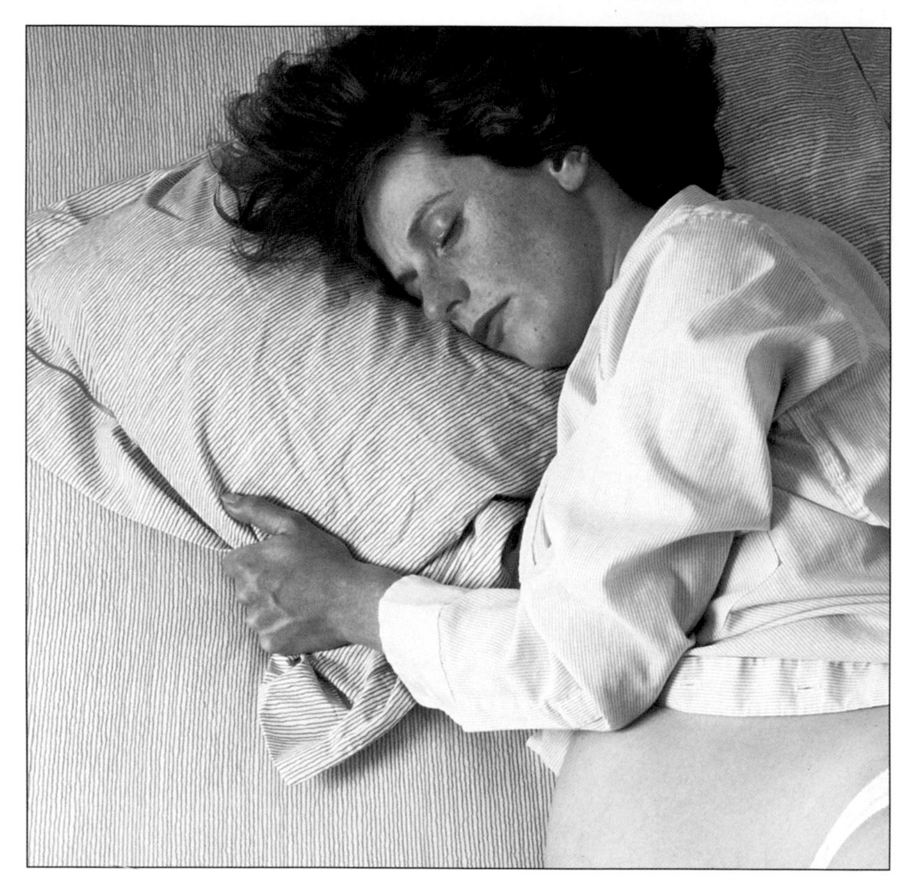

Some of the less pleasant side-effects of pregnancy, such as nausea and heartburn, may be relieved with the help of essential oils.

PREGNANCY

During pregnancy, there are certain oils that should not be used. See page 39.

HEARTBURN

This is a form of indigestion that seems particularly to afflict pregnant women. One drop of peppermint or sandalwood oil in water usually brings some relief.

MORNING SICKNESS

Peppermint oil has a very calming effect on the digestive system, and one drop in a glass of honey water should help with nausea. Peppermint tea may also bring some relief.

EPISIOTOMY

Many women have an episiotomy (a cut at the bottom of the vagina) during labor or a tear caused by pushing the baby out. Even if you have suffered neither of these, you may still be feeling very sore. Lavender oil in the bath is very soothing and also speeds up the healing process.

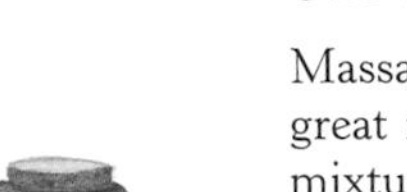

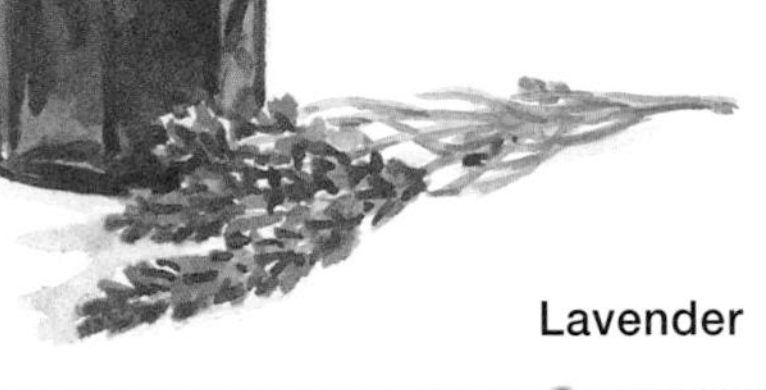

Lavender

LABOR

Massage of the lower back can bring great relief during a long labor. A mixture of 15 drops of lavender oil and 5 drops each of rose and ylang-ylang should also help relaxation and lift the spirits when you are feeling exhausted. Ask a partner, friend, or midwife to massage the lower back with firm, upward-sweeping strokes.

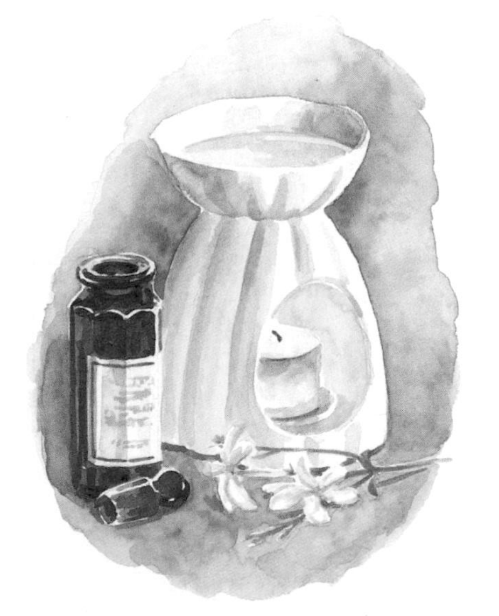

POSTNATAL DEPRESSION

On the third or fourth day after birth, the immense hormonal upheavals that are taking place in your body can cause postnatal depression. This can be eased with jasmine or ylang-ylang oil. Use them in the bath or on burners to scent the room.

Jasmine or ylang-ylang essential oils lift the spirits if you are coping with post-natal exhaustion and hormonal changes.

Aromatherapy oils can help relieve menopausal symptoms and allow you to enjoy your maturity to the full.

MENOPAUSE

The two most common problems women suffer during the menopause are hot flashes and mood swings or depression. Baths with 4 drops of clary sage oil and 2 each of peppermint and geranium are recommended. For hot flashes, try inhaling some peppermint oil on a tissue. A whole body massage using roughly equal proportions of geranium, sandalwood, and camomile oils should prove beneficial. Or you can use the same mixture to massage into your neck and throat.

SKIN AND HAIR

The skin readily absorbs essential oils, making them ideal for skin complaints. Many oils can be used in preparations that are cosmetic, too. Use lemon oil if you have oily skin, sandalwood for dry skin, and rose or frankincense for mature skin. When using essential oils on the face, you use a weaker dilution than that for the body (see page 22).

ACNE

Spots and acne are most commonly the result of either hormonal imbalance or poor diet – or both. Acne is particularly associated with adolescence, but in fact, spots can occur at any time, and many women get them just before menstruation whatever their age. Cutting out junk food and very spicy or fatty foods is imperative, and drinking plenty of spring water is important, too. Don't squeeze spots – this only encourages the sebaceous glands to produce more. Put 5 drops each of lemon, cypress, and juniper oils into 2 oz. (50ml) of water and mix well. Bathe the affected area with this several times a day. At night, you could use the same essential oils mixed in a carrier oil.

Adolescents often suffer from skin problems that may be relieved by antiseptic essential oils when used in combination with a healthy diet.

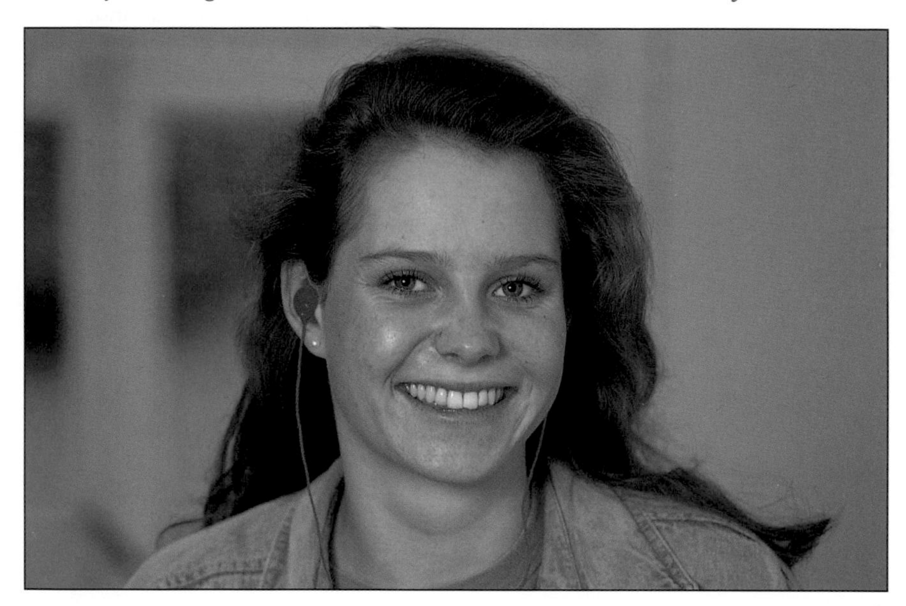

COLD SORES (HERPES SIMPLEX)

This very common virus brings blisters around the mouth that burst and sometimes bleed. *If the problem spreads or persists, consult your doctor.* Keep the affected area scrupulously clean, and wash it separately with sterile cotton. There should be no contact with any other parts of the face. Adults with cold sores should avoid children, for whom this can be a very painful condition.

Bergamot, eucalyptus, and tea tree are all suitable oils. Mix a combination of 2 or 3 of these in carrier oil and apply regularly to the affected area.

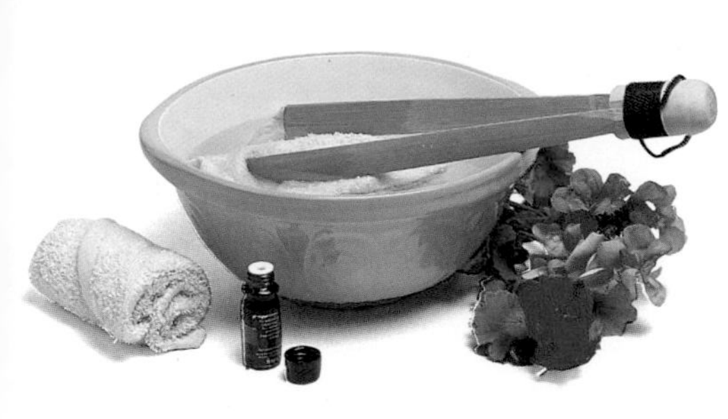

If eczema results in broken skin, massage is not advisable. Instead, use a compress of camomile, lavender, or geranium.

ECZEMA

Eczema can stem from a very wide range of causes. It is often hereditary, it can be an allergic reaction, and it can be triggered by stress or tiredness. I have suffered from eczema all my life, and at one time it was quite bad – my fingers were cracked, swollen, and bleeding. I find that plenty of rest (and relief from stress, if possible) combined with a sensible diet (no caffeine or alcohol) clears it up within a week. For localized relief, dab on pure lavender oil every hour and, providing it is a fairly mild attack, the skin heals over in 3–4 hours. This is not, however, recommended if the skin is very broken. Camomile, lavender, and geranium are all wonderfully healing and soothing for eczema, and juniper is good for "weeping" eczema. You can use these in the bath, as a compress, or as a general massage oil (in carrier oil), especially if your eczema is triggered by stress. *Do not, however, massage over any areas of broken skin.*

ATHLETE'S FOOT

Athlete's foot is caused by a fungal growth which thrives in the sort of conditions provided by sweaty socks! Wash the feet frequently and keep them exposed to the air whenever possible. You can dab pure lavender, lemon, or tea tree onto the affected area, or put any of these oils into a bowl of warm water as a foot bath. You could also use these essential oils in a carrier oil and apply to the whole area at bedtime.

RINGWORM

There is no worm involved in ringworm. It is a highly contagious fungal infection that forms a ring on the skin. Treat with 10 drops each of lavender and tea tree oils, and 5 drops of geranium in carrier oil and apply on cotton balls to the affected area regularly.

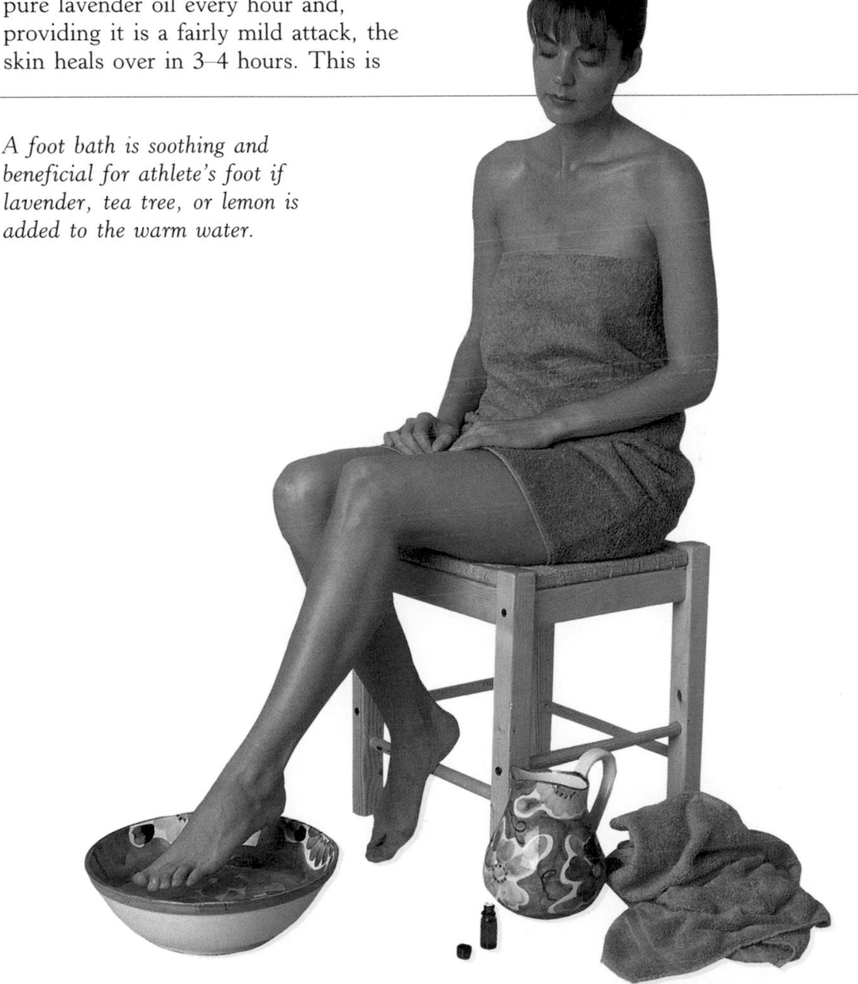

A foot bath is soothing and beneficial for athlete's foot if lavender, tea tree, or lemon is added to the warm water.

DANDRUFF

Dandruff can affect both dry and oily scalps, and it requires regular, frequent treatments before you will see an improvement. For an overnight treatment to use two or three times a week, blend 10 drops each of eucalyptus and rosemary oils and 5 drops of juniper or tea tree in 2 oz. (50ml) of carrier oil. Apply generously all over the hair and scalp and cover in plastic wrap. Next morning, shampoo thoroughly and use the same blend of essential oils in warm water (rather than carrier oil) as a final rinse.

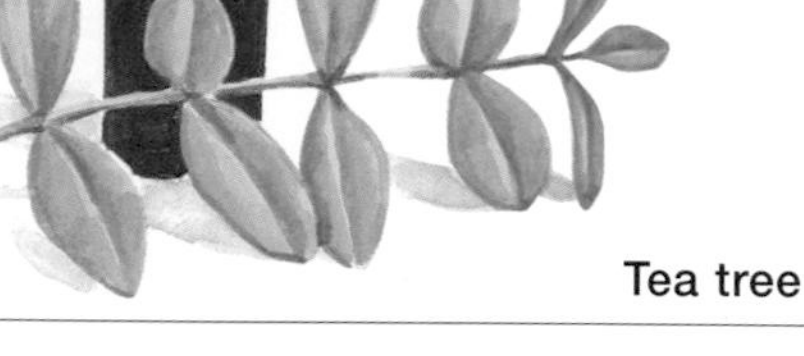

Tea tree

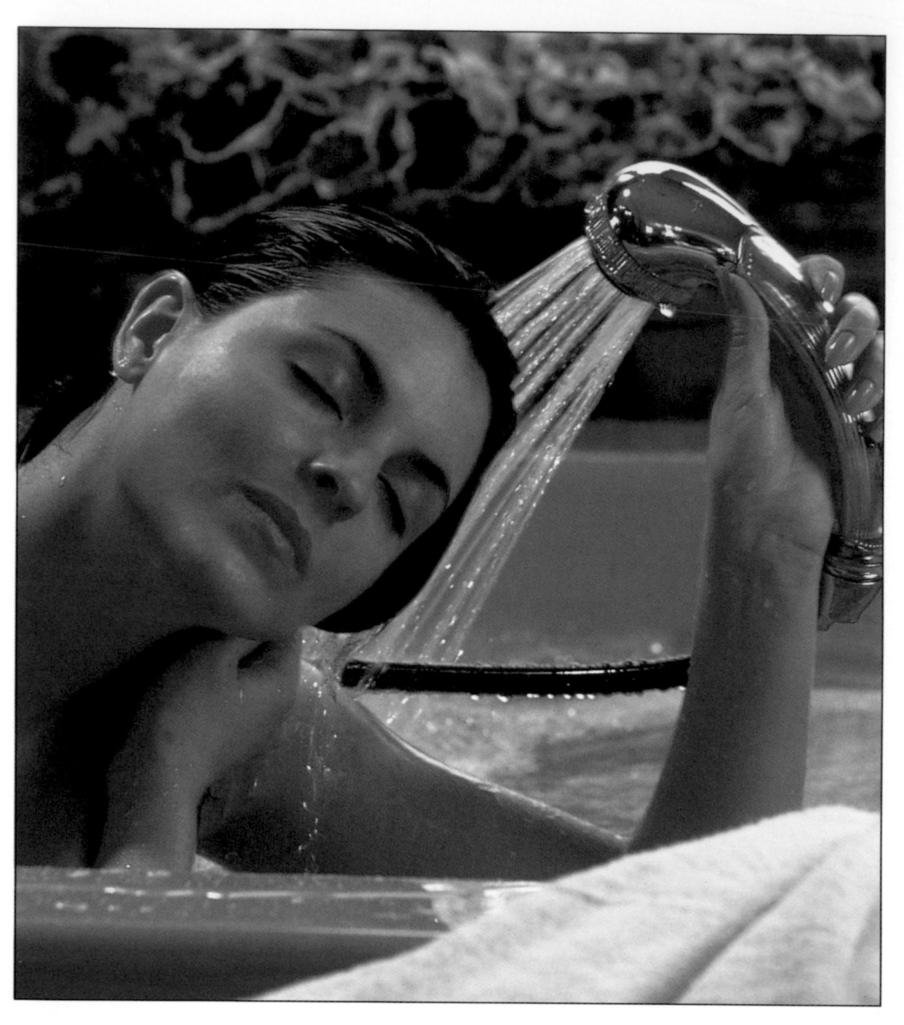

Aromatherapy oils may be very beneficial for problems affecting the hair and scalp, including dandruff, hair loss, and head lice.

HEAD LICE

Outbreaks of head lice are not uncommon in schools. The head louse lays its eggs at the base of the hair shaft and can cause discomfort and even infection of the scalp. Massage a blend of 6 drops of rosemary or tea tree oil, 5 of eucalyptus or geranium, and 6 of lavender in 2 oz. (50ml) of carrier oil into the scalp. The hair should be completely covered, then wrapped in a towel or in plastic wrap. The mixture can be left on for up to 2 hours. Comb through and wash the hair thoroughly (you will need a lot of shampoo to get rid of all the oil). Repeat on a daily basis until the problem has cleared up.

HAIR LOSS

Hair loss can be sudden and temporary – after giving birth, as a result of shock or stress, as a side-effect to illness or drugs – or it can be simple male-pattern baldness. In the former cases, the following massage oil will encourage regrowth. In the latter, it may help to slow down the inevitable.

Mix 10 drops each of rosemary and lavender oils plus 5 drops of sandalwood in carrier oil, and massage deeply into the scalp. Leave on for at least an hour, then shampoo.

CHILDREN'S PROBLEMS

Children respond very quickly to essential oils and require much weaker doses than adults. As a general rule, do not give children under 10 any oil to be taken internally and, for children over 10, halve the adult dose. With oils to be applied externally, halve the adult dose for children over 5. For younger children and babies, it should be only a quarter of the adult dose. Use only the oils listed here or on page 16 or 39.

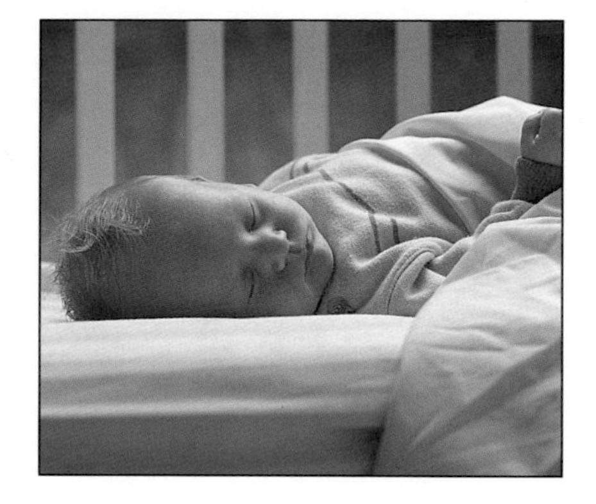

A drop of lavender on the pillow will promote a deeper sleep.

SLEEP PROBLEMS

A drop of lavender on the quilt will help a baby or child to sleep. If a cold and a stuffy nose is preventing sleep, a drop of eucalyptus will clear the head. *Never apply these to the child's skin, only to the bedding.*

COLIC

Young babies often suffer a bout of stomach pain, known as colic, at a regular time every day, often, though not always, in the early evening. A warm camomile compress is very soothing, and often the baby will fall asleep with it on. Make a compress by soaking a cloth in warm water with 1 drop of camomile oil. Squeeze out the water and lay it over the baby's stomach, then cover with a blanket. Do the same for young children with stomachaches.

DIAPER RASH

If your baby has severe, long-lasting diaper rash, it may be because an infection has set in, and *in this case you should consult your doctor*. If it seems to be a mild case, however, put 1 drop of lavender oil in the baby's bath. If the skin is not broken, you could also apply a mixture of 4 drops of lavender and 2 of camomile in 2 oz. (50ml) of carrier oil. You will need only a tiny amount at a time, and of course, you should apply it very gently. You could also use this mixture as a preventative.

TEARS AND TANTRUMS

Young children are extremely prone to tears and tantrums, whether from frustration or nerves. A drop of lavender, clary sage, or geranium oil, preferably in the bath or, alternatively, on their clothes, can often calm them.

TEETHING

A drop of lavender or camomile oil on the baby's pajamas or bedding will be calming and soothing.

FIRST AID

There are some oils that may bring instant relief in minor emergencies. If symptoms persist, however, or for more severe accidents, always consult a doctor or hospital.

These are some of the occasions when pure oils may be applied. The most useful oil is lavender, and it is a good idea always to take a bottle with you on vacation as it may alleviate a whole variety of problems – burns, scalds, cuts, and sunburn. It can also help with sleeplessness and minor headaches. (See also First Aid on page 15.)

BURNS AND SCALDS

Depending on the size of the affected area, dab on pure lavender, tea tree, or eucalyptus oil on a cotton swab: or submerge the area in cold water to which 10 drops of one of the above oils has been added; or apply a compress with one of these oils. *Serious burns or scalds must be treated by a doctor.*

TOOTHACHE

A drop of clove oil on a cotton swab can be applied directly to the tooth and usually brings fairly rapid relief.

Peppermint oil can also give some relief. Neither, however, is a cure, so you should visit your dentist as soon as possible.

Peppermint

INSECT STINGS

If an insect sting has been left behind, remove it with tweezers. Then apply 1 drop of pure tea tree or lavender oil on a cotton swab. You can repeat this process (alternating the oils or mixing them together) until you can see or feel an improvement. *If you are allergic to insect stings, and an increasing number of people seem to be, see a doctor immediately.*

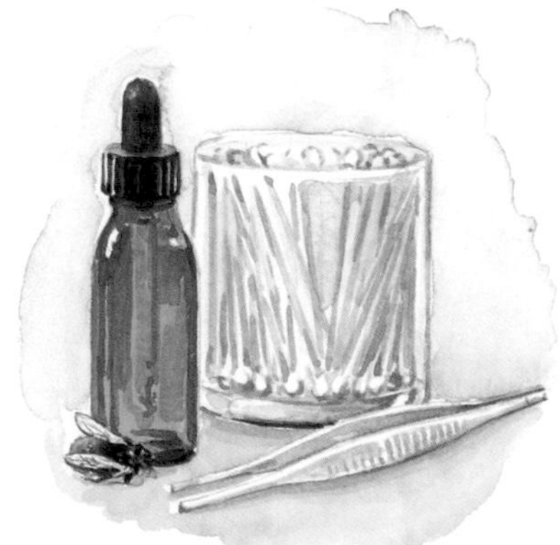

Remove the insect sting with tweezers, if necessary, and dab on pure tea tree or lavender oil.

WOUNDS, CUTS, AND GRAZES

For minor wounds, cuts, and grazes, you can apply pure lavender or tea tree oil. They can also be applied as compresses or added to a bath.

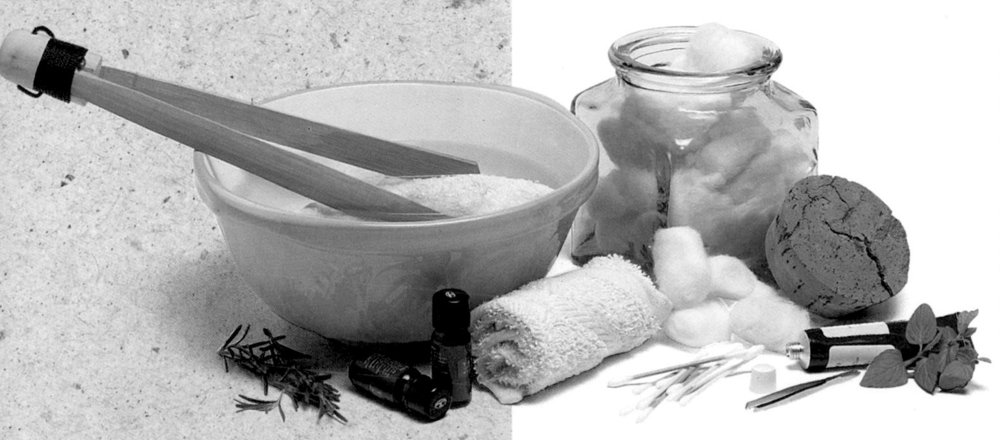

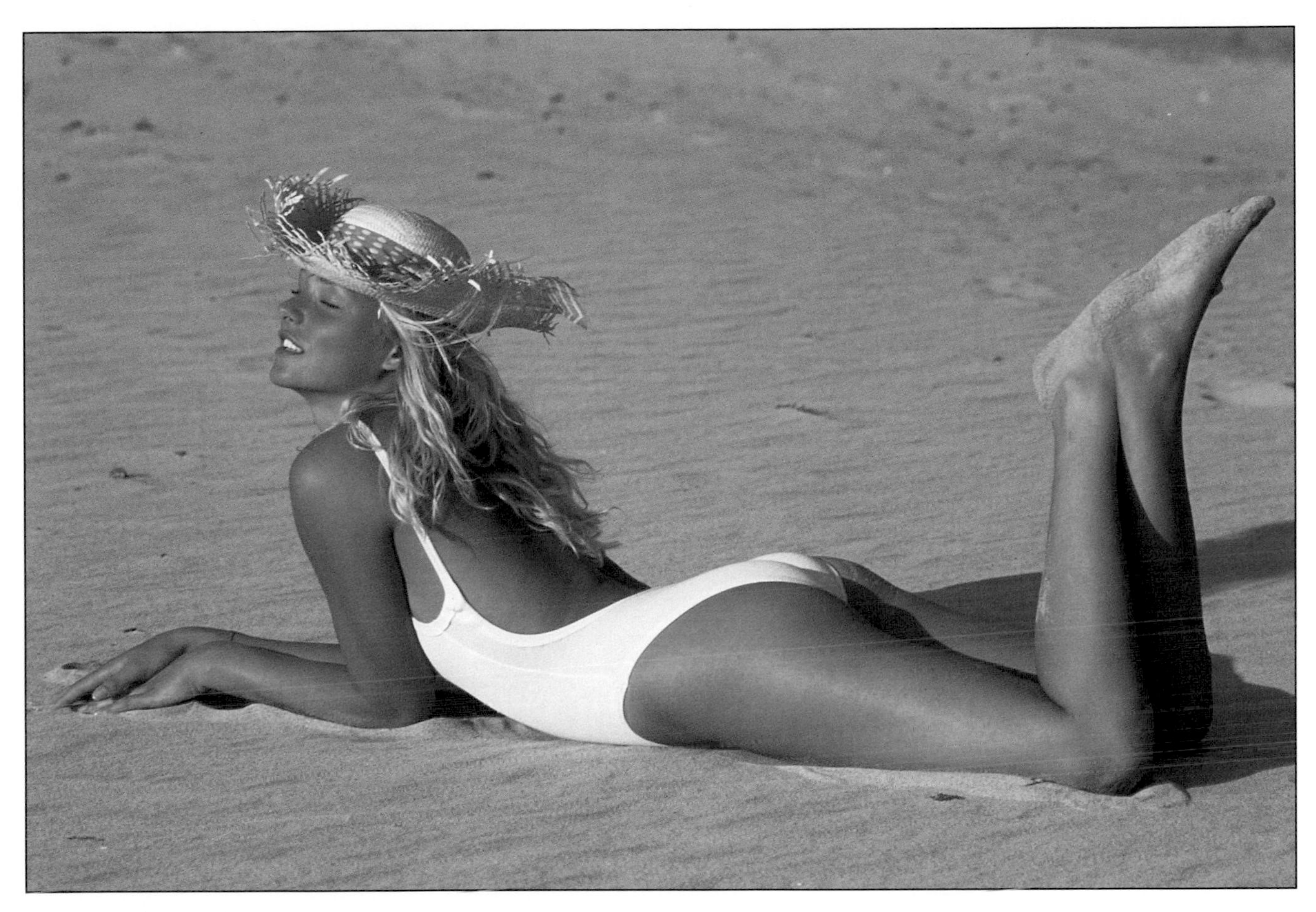

Always use a very high protection suncream when sunbathing, and cover up sensitive areas like the face and the shoulders at the first sign of trouble. If you get sunburned, soaking in a lavender or peppermint bath will bring some relief.

SUNBURN

If the area is not too inflamed, you can dab on pure lavender oil. For a larger, more sensitive area, add lavender or peppermint oil to a tepid bath and soak in it for at least 20 minutes.

SPRAINS

If in doubt about any sort of injury, consult a doctor or the emergency room in a hospital. If you know it is only a minor sprain or as an interim measure, apply a cold compress using a bowl of water with 3 drops each of eucalyptus, lavender, and rosemary oils added. Replace as the compress warms up.

BRUISES

For a minor bruise, apply repeated compresses with a cloth soaked in a bowl of water to which 4 drops each of fennel and marjoram oils have been added. Arnica ointment, available from health food stores, is also excellent for bruises, and if applied immediately, it can sometimes stop them from appearing altogether. Arnica is also available in pill form.

Consulting an Aromatherapist

If you decide to consult an aromatherapist, you must always be sure to find one who is professionally qualified (see opposite). It is also a good idea, if possible, to have a personal recommendation from someone whose opinion you trust. This way, you will also know what to expect when you go for a consultation, as different therapists use different techniques. The most important priority, though, is that there is a feeling of empathy between you and your therapist. If you feel uncomfortable in any way, then this is not the therapist for you.

A professional aromatherapist is particularly useful if you have a specific condition that you feel needs qualified help, or if you want a course of treatment – particularly for massage. One of the key areas for aromatherapists is stress, and the very relaxing treatment of a massage with the right essential oils can be of enormous benefit in stress-related problems.

For a first appointment, allow between 1½ and 2 hours. Subsequently, the sessions will probably drop to just 1 hour, but the first time, the therapist may want to discuss your physical and emotional health in some depth.

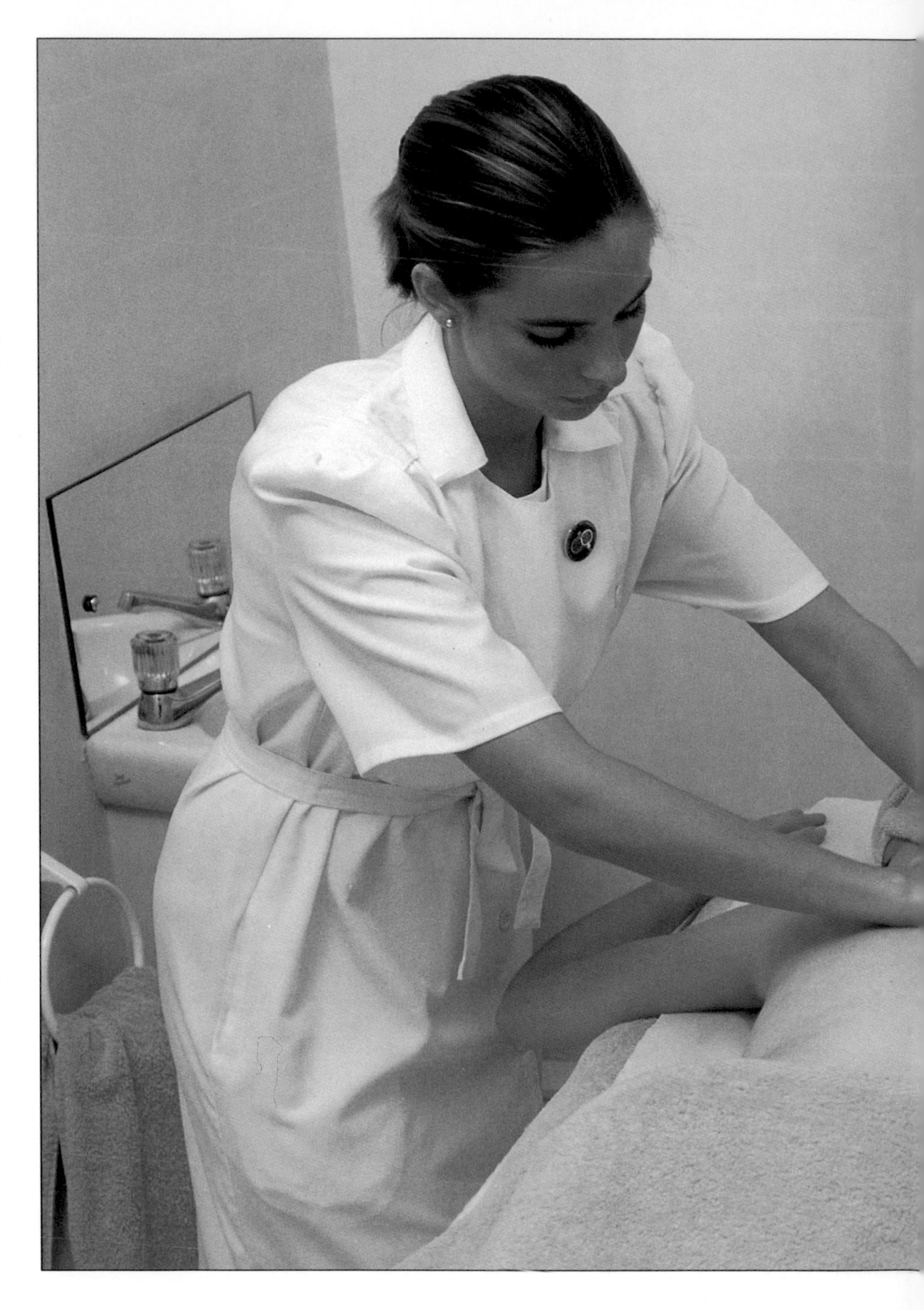

A professional massage from a qualified aromatherapist is a real treat, particularly if you are suffering from stress or any related problems.

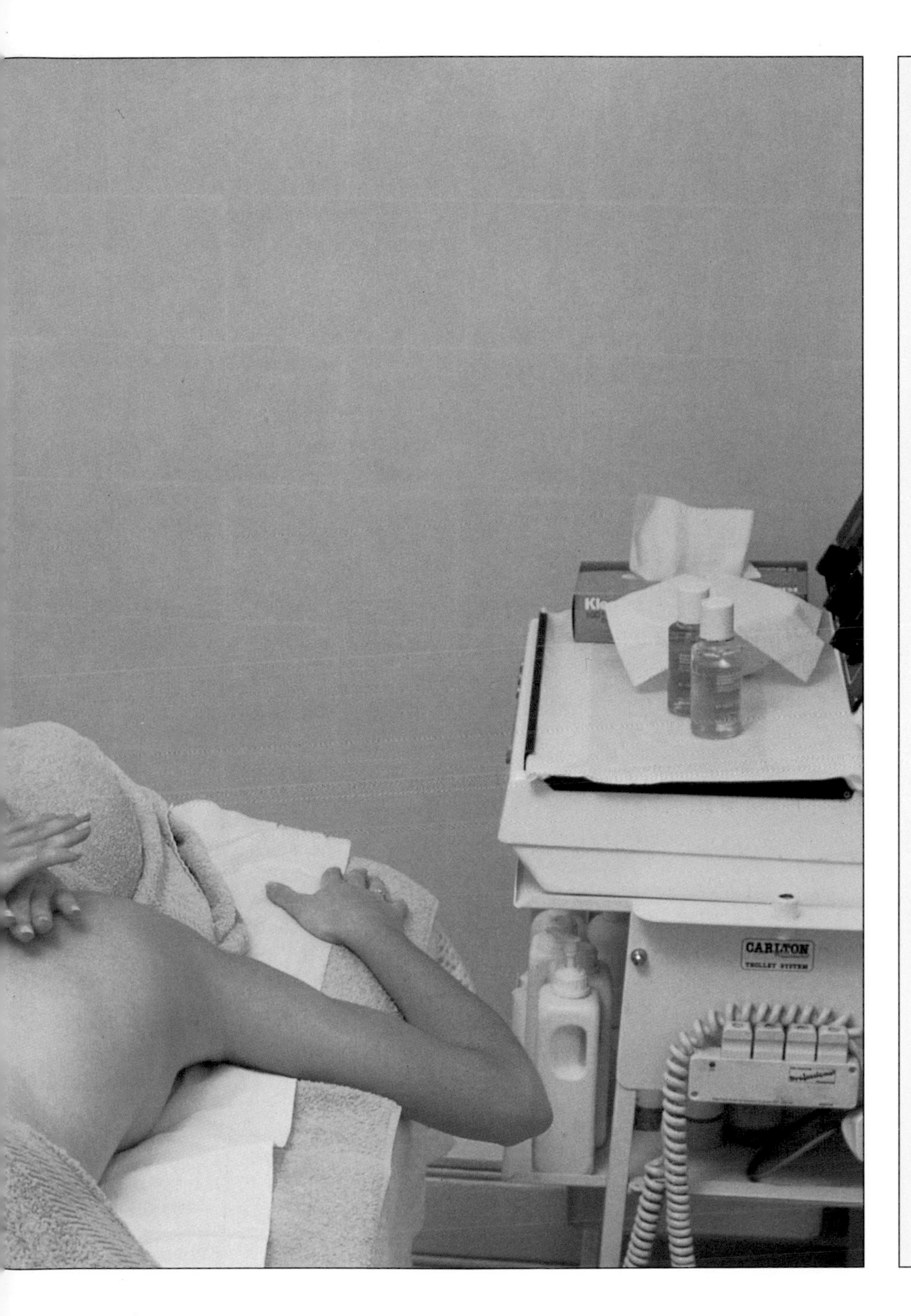

Useful Adresses

Professional associations –
Natural Association for Holistic Aromatherapy
P.O. Box 17622
Boulder, CO 80308
Tel: 800-566-6735

Mail order: essential oils –
Avalon Natural Cosmetics
1105 Industrial Ave
Petaluna, CA 94952
Tel: 707-769-5120

Directories: practitioners –
Holistic Health Directory & Resource Guide
42 Pleasant St
Watertown, MA 02172
Tel: 617-926-0200

Check the Yellow Pages for local suppliers and practitioners.

Reading List

Shirley Price, *Practical Aromatherapy* Thorsons, 1983.
Maggie Tisserand, *Aromatherapy for Women* Thorsons, 1983.
Robert Tisserand, *The Art of Aromatherapy* Daniel, 1977.
Dr. Jean Valnet, *The Practice of Aromatherapy* Daniel, 1982.

INDEX

Note: Page numbers in *italics* refer to illustrations

abdomen, massage 36, *36*
acne 10, 12, 15, 16, 19, 39, 54
addresses, useful 61
air freshener 18
alcohol 55
Alexander technique 47
almond oil *22*, 52
anemia 18
ankles, massage 37, *37*
antidepressants *see* depression
antiseptics 11, 12, 13, 14, 15, 16, 19, 43
anxiety 9, 12, 13, 40
aphrodisiacs 10, 11, 19
appetite, loss of 18
apricot kernel oil 22
arms, massage 35, *35*
arnica 15, 59
aromatherapist, consulting 60
arthritis 12, 13, 14, 15, 16, 18, 21, 39, 46
asthma 10, 15, 19, 45
athlete's foot 15, 19, 55
Australian aborigines 15
Avicenna 4

Bach flower remedy 15
back, massage 32-3, *32-3*
backache/pain 12, 46, 47
basil 11, *11*, 20
baths 19, 21
benzoin 14
bergamot 12, *12*, 41, 45, *45*, 52, 54
  cautions 8
bites 10, 11, 12, 15
blisters 15
blood
  purifying 14
  staunching flow 12
blood pressure
  high 6, 11, 15, 48
  low 48

breast milk, increasing 10, 15
bronchitis 11, 12, 13, 14, 15, 16, 17, 19, 39, 45
bruising 15, 19, 59
bunions 18
burns 4-5, 10, 11, 15, 16, 20, 39, 58
buttocks, massage 31, *31*

caffeine 55
calendula oil *22*
calluses 18
camomile 12, 16, 46, 47, 49, 51, 53, 55, 57
camphor 18
canker sores 15, 49
cardamon 19, *19*
carrier oils *22*
catarrh 13, 18, 19, 44
cautions 8
cedarwood 13, 45
cell renewal 13
cellulite 12, 15, 19, 52
  massaging *52*
chest
  infections of 21
  massage *45*
chickenpox 16
childbirth 39, 53
children
  calming 9
  oils suitable for 39
  problems 39, 57
  starter pack for 16
circulation 11, 12, 14, 18, 48
  problems 8, 39
citronella 19
citrus oils 23
  cautions 8
clary sage 9, *9*, 12, 16, 21, 23, 40, *40*, 41, 44, 51, 53, 57
clove 14, *14*, 58
coconut oil *22*
cold sores (see herpes simplex)
colds 10, 11, 13, 14, 15, 16, 17, 18, 19, 20, 38, 43
colic 15, 16, 18, 57
compresses 14, 39, 45, *45*, 50, 57, 59
  technique 21
congestion 18, 20
constipation 12, 15, 18, 49, 50
contra-indications 24, 39
convulsions 16
corns 18
cosmetics 4, 54
coughs 10, 11, 12, 13, 14, 15, 17, 38, 43
cramps 47
  menstrual 39, 51
Crusaders 4
cupping 28, *28*
cuts 13, 20, 58
cypress 12, *12*, 43, 48, *48*, 54
cystitis 11, 12, 13, 14, 15, 18, 51

dandruff 13, 39, 56
decongestants 14, 43
deodorants 17, 18, 19
depression 9, 11, 12, 19, 38, 39, 41, 53
dermatitis 13, 14
diaper rash 15, 16, 57
diarrhea 10, 11, 16, 18, 50
digestive problems 11, 16, 18, 38, 39, 49-50
digestive system 15
diuretics 11, 14, 15

earache 16, 45
eczema 10, 11, 12, 13, 16, 19, 39, 55
effleurage *26*, *26*
Egypt 4, *5*
emotional problems 39, 40-2
episiotomy 53
essential oils 4
  blending 23
  buying 6, *22*
  cautions 8
  contra-indications 39
  dilutions *22*
  distillation 4, *5*
  internal use 21, *21*
  storing *8*, *22*, *22*
  using 6, *22*-3
  using neat 20
eucalyptus 14, *14*, 15, 16, 20, 21, 43, *43*,

44, 45, 46, 47, 51, 54, 56, 57, 58, 59
  extracting essence *4*
exhaustion 19

facial toner 9
fatigue 18, 40
feet
  bathing *55*
  massage 37, *37*
fennel 12, 15, *15*, 59
fever 18
first aid 15, 38, 39, 58-9
flatulence 14, 15, 17, 18, 49
flu 13, 14, 16, 17, 18, 19, 43
fluid retention 14, 16, 17, 19
foot baths *55*
frankincense 4, 13, 45, 46, 54
fungal infections 15

gargles 21, 43, 44
Gattefosse, Rene-Maurice 4-5
geranium 10, *10*, 16, 40, 49, 50, *50*, 51, 53, 55, 56, 57
  extracting essence *4*
ginger 12, 44, 46, 47, 49
gout 14
grapefruit 19, *19*
grapeseed oil *22*
grazes 39, 58
Greece 4
gum benjamin 14

hacking 28, *28*
hair
  care 17
  loss 56
  oily 13, 19
  problems 39, 56
halitosis 12
hands, massage 35, *35*
hangovers 39, 50
hayfever 11
head, massage *42*
head lice 39, 56
headaches 11, 14, 15, 16, 17, 19, 21, 42
heart 11, 18
heartburn 39, 53
hemorrhoids 12, 18, 48
herbal teas 49
herpes simplex 14, 15, 54
hiccups 15, 16
holistic medicine 5
honey water 49, 51, 53
  making *21*
hot flushes 53
hyssop 19, *19*
hysteria 9

immune system 10, 17
incense 4, 14
indigestion 14, 15, 49
  heartburn 39, 53
infections 10, 14
  minor 19
inhalations 14, 20, 21, *44*
insect bites and stings 10, 12, 15, 58
insect repellents 12, 14, 15, 17, 18, 19
insomnia 9, 11, 12, 15, 16, 17, 21, 38, 39

jasmine 10, *10*, 21, 41, 53
joints, swollen 12
juniper 14, 43, 46, 47, 48, 50, 51, 52, 54, 55, 56

kidney stones 10, 15
kidneys 14
kneading 27, *27*

labor pains 10, 53
laryngitis 11, 13, 44
lavender 5, 11, *11*, 12, 15, 16, 20, 21, 40, 41, 42, 43, 44, 45, 46, 47, 48, 49, 50, 51, 52, 53, *53*, 55, 56, 57, 58, 59
legs, massage 29-30, *29-30*, 37, *37*
lemon 10, *10*, 12, 41, 44, 46, 48, 49, 54, 55
  cautions 8
lemon balm *see* melissa
lime 48
liver 16
lymphatic system 6

Magi 4
mandarin 16, *16*
  cautions 8
marjoram 12, 15, *15*, 42, 46, 47, *47*, 48, 50, 51, 59
massage 5, *6-7*
  basic strokes 26-8, *26-8*
  basic technique 20, *20*
  contra-indications 24
  full body routine 29-37
  preparation for 24, 25
  professional 60, *60-1*
  purpose 24
  resting after 24
medicine, essences used for 4
melissa 17, *17*, 40, 42
menopause 53
menstrual problems 9, 11, 13, 17
  cramps 15, 39, 51
  fluid retention 14
migraine 15, 16, 19, 42
mind, sharpening and focusing 19
morning sickness 39, 53
mosquito repellent 14
mouthwashes 21, 49
muscular problems 11, 12, 15, 16, 18, 38, 39, 46, 46-8, 47
myrrh 4, 13, *13*, 52

nails, brittle 10
nausea 12, 15, 16, 17, 49
  morning sickness 39, 53
neck, massage 34, *34*
neroli 9, 23, 40, 41, 52
nervous exhaustion 17, 18, 19, 40
nervous stress/tension 17, 19
nettle stings 58
nose bleeds 12

obesity 15, 16
olfactory system 5, 6
olive oil *22*
orange 17, *17*, 41, 48
  cautions 8
orange blossom *see* neroli
osteoarthritis 46
painkillers 11
palpitations 16

patchouli 19, 40
peach kernel oil *22*
pepper, black 18, *18*, 48, 50
peppermint 15, 16, *16*, 21, 40, 42, 43, 44, 49, 50, 53, 58, *58*, 59
perfume notes *23*
petitgrain 17, *17*
petrissage *27*, *27*
pillows, oils on 21, *21*
pine 18, *18*, 46
PMS (premenstrual syndrome) 9, 15, 39, 51
post-natal depression 10, 53
pregnancy
  contra-indications 39
  treatment during 39, 52-3
premenstrual syndrome *see* PMS
psoriasis 12

rejuvenation 11
relaxation starter pack 9-11
"Rescue Remedy" 15
respiratory problems 11, 12, 13, 14, 18, 21, 39, 43-5
rheumatism 11, 12, 13, 14, 15, 16, 18, 21, 39, 46
ringworm 15, 16, 55
Rome 4
room scents 19, *21*, *21*
rose 11, 16, 40, 41, 50, 53, 54
rosemary 13, *13*, 15, 21, 40, 46, 47, *47*, 48, 50, 52, 56, 59
  extracting essence *4*
rosewood 17

sage 9
sandalwood 11, *11*, 12, *23*, 40, 44, 48, 50, 51, 53, 54, 56
scabies 16
scalds 16, 58
sedatives 10, 11, 14, 16
shock 9, 15
shoulders, massage 34, *34*
sinuses 18, 21
sinusitis 10, 11, 16, 44
skin
  absorption through 5, 6
  care 17
  chapped 19
  cracked 19
  dry 11, *22*, 54
  infections 15
  itchiness 16
  mature 13, *22*, 54
  oily 12, 13, 17, 19, 54
  problems 9, 10, 11, 12, 13, 14, 39, 54-5
  rejuvenation 13
  toning 9
sleep problems
  see also insomnia
  in children 16, 57
smell, sense of 6
sports injuries 46
spots 15
sprains 12, 15, 18, 21, 59
steam inhalations 14, 20, *44*
  method 21
stings 11, 15, 20, 39, 58
stomachaches 16
stomach upsets 16
strains 15
stress 9, 12, 13, 19, 38, 39, 40-2
stretchmarks 13, 16, 52
sunburn 11, 59
sunlight, oils dangerous in 8, 10, 12, 17
swellings 21

tagetes 18, *18*
tantrums 16, 57
tea tree 12, 15, 16, 43, 44, 49, 50, 52, 54, 55, 56, *56*, 58
techniques, basic 20-1
teething 16, 57
tension 7, 11, 15, 40
therapeutic starter pack 12-14
throat
  infections of 10, 21, 44
  massage *45*
  sore 11, 12, 15, 39, 43, 44
Tisserand, Robert 5
tissues, oils on 21
tonsilitis 12, 45
toothache 16, 58
trauma 15
travel sickness 12, 16
Tutankhamum 4

uric acid, expelling 14
urinary infections 14, 18

vaporization 19, 21
varicose veins 12, 48
vetiver 10
vomiting 15, 16, 17

wheatgerm oil *22*, *52*
women's problems 39, 51-3
  see also menstrual problems
wounds 12, 13, 14, 15, 19, 58
wrist, massage 35, *35*

yeast 12, 13, 15, 52
ylang-ylang 9, *9*, 40, 41, 48, 51, 53
yoga 47

AKNOWLEDGMENTS

The author would like to dedicate this book to Christian.

Quarto would like to thank the following people who supplied photographs:

Key: a=above b=below l=left r=right

E.T. Archive 5; Ken Scott/Tony Stone Images 7; Harry Smith Horticultural Collection 9, 10, 12(a), 13(al), 14(a), 17(a), 18(al), 19(a); Mauritius/Ace 41; Pictor 43; Tibor Bognor/Ace 46; Chris Harvey/Tony Stone Images 47; Nawrocki Stock Photos/Ace 48; David Le Lossy/Image Bank 50(a); Romilly Lockyer/Image Bank 52(b); Simon Wilkinson/Image Bank 53; Pictor 54; Gabe Palmer/Ace 56; Auschromes/Ace 57(a); David Le Lossy/Image Bank 58; James Wedge/Tony Stone Images 60.

Quarto would like to thank the Tisserand Institute for their assistance.